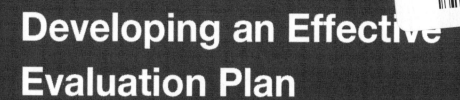

# Developing an Effective Evaluation Plan

**Setting the course for
effective program evaluation**

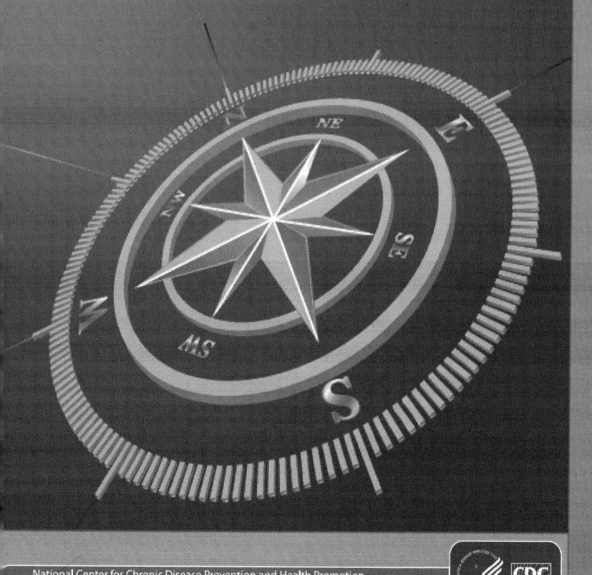

National Center for Chronic Disease Prevention and Health Promotion

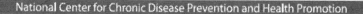
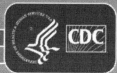

# Acknowledgments

This workbook was developed by the Centers for Disease Control and Prevention's (CDC's) Office on Smoking and Health (OSH) and Division of Nutrition, Physical Activity, and Obesity (DNPAO). This workbook was developed as part of a series of technical assistance workbooks for use by program managers, and evaluators. The workbooks are intended to offer guidance and facilitate capacity building on a wide range of evaluation topics. We encourage users to adapt the tools and resources in this workbook to meet their program's evaluation needs.

This workbook applies the CDC Framework for Program Evaluation in Public Health (http://www.cdc.gov/eval/framework/index.htm). The Framework lays out a six-step process for the decisions and activities involved in conducting an evaluation. While the Framework provides steps for program evaluation, the steps are not always linear and represent a more back-and-forth effort; some can be completed concurrently. In some cases, it makes more sense to skip a step and come back to it. The important thing is that the steps are considered within the specific context of your program.

Suggested Citation: Developing an Effective Evaluation Plan. Atlanta, Georgia: Centers for Disease Control and Prevention, National Center for Chronic Disease Prevention and Health Promotion, Office on Smoking and Health; Division of Nutrition, Physical Activity, and Obesity, 2011.

# Table of Contents

# Figures

# Acronyms

| | |
|---|---|
| **BRFSS** | Behavioral Risk Factor Surveillance System |
| **CDC** | Centers for Disease Control and Prevention |
| **DNPAO** | Division of Nutrition, Physical Activity, and Obesity |
| **ESW** | Evaluation Stakeholder Workgroup |
| **NIDRR** | National Institute on Disability and Rehabilitation Research |
| **OSH** | Office on Smoking and Health |
| **PRAMS** | Pregnancy Risk Assessment Monitoring System |
| **YRBS** | Youth Risk Behavior Surveillance |

# Part I: Developing Your Evaluation Plan

## WHO IS THE AUDIENCE FOR THIS WORKBOOK?

The purpose of this workbook is to help public health program managers, administrators, and evaluators develop a joint understanding of what constitutes an evaluation plan, why it is important, and how to develop an effective evaluation plan in the context of the planning process. This workbook is intended to assist in developing an evaluation plan but is not intended to serve as a complete resource on *how to implement* program evaluation. Rather, it is intended to be used along with other evaluation resources, such as those listed in the Resource Section of this workbook. The workbook was written by the staff of the Office on Smoking and Health (OSH) and the Division of Nutrition, Physical Activity, and Obesity (DNPAO) at the Centers for Disease Control and Prevention (CDC). However, the content and steps for writing an evaluation plan can be applied to any public health program or initiative. Part I of this workbook defines and describes how to write an effective evaluation plan. Part II of this workbook includes exercises, worksheets, tools, and a Resource Section to facilitate program staff and evaluation stakeholder workgroup (ESW) thinking through the concepts presented in Part I of this workbook.

## WHAT IS AN EVALUATION PLAN?

An evaluation plan is a written document that describes how you will monitor and evaluate your program, as well as how you intend to use evaluation results for program improvement and decision making. The evaluation plan clarifies how you will describe the *"What,"* the *"How,"* and the *"Why It Matters"* for your program.

> An evaluation plan is a written document that describes how you will monitor and evaluate your program, so that you will be able to describe the *"What"*, the *"How"*, and the *"Why It Matters"* for your program and use evaluation results for program improvement and decision making.

- The *"What"* reflects the description of your program and how its activities are linked with the intended effects. It serves to clarify the program's purpose and anticipated outcomes.

- The *"How"* addresses the process for implementing a program and provides information about whether the program is operating with fidelity to the program's design. Additionally, the "How" (or process evaluation), along with output and/or short-term outcome information, helps clarify if changes should be made during implementation.

- The *"Why It Matters"* provides the rationale for your program and the impact it has on public health. This is also sometimes referred to as the "so what" question. Being able to demonstrate that your program has made a difference is critical to program sustainability.

An evaluation plan is similar to a roadmap. It clarifies the steps needed to assess the processes and outcomes of a program. An effective evaluation plan is more than a column of indicators added to your program's work plan. It is a dynamic tool (i.e., a "living document") that should be updated on an ongoing basis to reflect program changes and priorities over time. An evaluation plan serves as a bridge between evaluation and program planning by highlighting program goals, clarifying measurable program objectives, and linking program activities with intended outcomes.

## WHY DO YOU WANT AN EVALUATION PLAN?

Just as using a roadmap facilitates progress on a long journey, an evaluation plan can clarify what direction your evaluation should take based on priorities, resources, time, and skills needed to accomplish the evaluation. The process of developing an evaluation plan in cooperation with an evaluation workgroup of stakeholders will foster collaboration and a sense of shared purpose. Having a *written evaluation plan* will foster transparency and ensure that stakeholders are on the same page with regards to the purpose, use, and users of the evaluation results. Moreover, use of evaluation results is not something that can be hoped or wished for but must be planned, directed, and intentional (Patton, 2008). A written plan is one of your most effective tools in your evaluation tool box.

A written evaluation plan can—

- create a shared understanding of the purpose(s), use, and users of the evaluation results,
- foster program transparency to stakeholders and decision makers,
- increase buy-in and acceptance of methods,
- connect multiple evaluation activities—this is especially useful when a program employs different contractors or contracts,
- serve as an advocacy tool for evaluation resources based on negotiated priorities and established stakeholder and decision maker information needs,
- help to identify whether there are sufficient program resources and time to accomplish desired evaluation activities and answer prioritized evaluation questions,
- assist in facilitating a smoother transition when there is staff turnover,
- facilitate evaluation capacity building among partners and stakeholders,

- provide a multi-year comprehensive document that makes explicit everything from stakeholders to dissemination to use of results, and
- facilitate good evaluation practice.

There are several critical elements needed to ensure that your evaluation plan lives up to its potential. These elements include ensuring (1) that your plan is collaboratively developed with a stakeholder workgroup, (2) that it is responsive to program changes and priorities, (3) that it covers multiple years if your project is ongoing, and (4) that it addresses your entire program rather than focusing on just one funding source or objective/activity. You will, by necessity, focus the evaluation based on feasibility, stage of development, ability to consume information, and other priorities that will be discussed in Steps 3 and 4 in this workbook. However, during the planning phase, your entire program should be considered by the evaluation group.

## HOW DO YOU WRITE AN EVALUATION PLAN?

This workbook is organized by describing the elements of the evaluation plan within the context of using the CDC's Framework for Program Evaluation in Public Health (http://www.cdc.gov/eval/) and the planning process. The elements of an evaluation plan that will be discussed in this workbook include:

- **Title page:** Contains an easily identifiable program name, dates covered, and basic focus of the evaluation.

- **Intended use and users:** Fosters transparency about the purpose(s) of the evaluation and identifies who will have access to evaluation results. It is important to build a market for evaluation results from the beginning. Clarifying the primary intended users, the members of the stakeholder evaluation workgroup, and the purpose(s) of the evaluation will help to build this market.

- **Program description:** Provides the opportunity for building a shared understanding of the theory of change driving the program. This section often includes a logic model and a description of the stage of development of the program in addition to a narrative description.

- **Evaluation focus:** Provides the opportunity to document how the evaluation focus will be narrowed and the rationale for the prioritization process. Given that there are never enough resources or time to answer every evaluation question, it is critical to work collaboratively to prioritize the evaluation based on a shared understanding of the theory of change identified in the logic model, the stage of development of the program, the intended uses of the evaluation, as well as feasibility issues. This section should delineate the criteria for evaluation prioritization and include a discussion of feasibility and efficiency.

- **Methods:** Identifies evaluation indicators and performance measures, data sources and methods, as well as roles and responsibilities. This section provides a clear description of how the evaluation will be implemented to ensure credibility of evaluation information.

- **Analysis and interpretation plan:** Clarifies how information will be analyzed and describes the process for interpretation of results. This section describes who will get to see interim results, whether there will be a stakeholder interpretation meeting or meetings, and methods that will be used to analyze the data.

- **Use, dissemination, and sharing plan:** Describes plans for use of evaluation results and dissemination of evaluation findings. Clear, specific plans for evaluation use should be discussed from the beginning. This section should include a broad overview of how findings are to be used as well as more detailed information about the intended modes and methods for sharing results with stakeholders. This is a critical but often neglected section of the evaluation plan.

## WHAT ARE THE KEY STEPS IN DEVELOPING AN EVALUATION PLAN USING CDC'S FRAMEWORK FOR PROGRAM EVALUATION?

CDC's Framework for Program Evaluation in Public Health (1999) is a guide to effectively evaluate public health programs and use the findings for program improvement and decision making. While the framework is described in terms of steps, the actions are not always linear and are often completed in a back-and-forth effort that is cyclical in nature. Similar to the framework, the development of an evaluation plan is an ongoing process. You may need to revisit a step during the process and complete other discrete steps concurrently. Within each step of the framework, there are important components that are useful to consider in the creation of an evaluation plan.

Figure 1: CDC Framework for Program Evaluation in Public Health

Steps:

1. Engage stakeholders.
2. Describe the program.
3. Focus the evaluation design.
4. Gather credible evidence.
5. Justify conclusions.
6. Ensure use and share lessons learned.

In addition to CDC's Framework for Program Evaluation in Public Health there are evaluation standards that will enhance the quality of evaluations by guarding against potential mistakes or errors in practice. The evaluation standards are grouped around four important attributes: utility, feasibility, propriety, and accuracy as indicated by the inner circle in Figure 1.

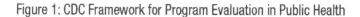

CDC's Framework for Program Evaluation

- **Utility:** Serve information needs of intended users.
- **Feasibility:** Be realistic, prudent, diplomatic, and frugal.
- **Propriety:** Behave legally, ethically, and with due regard for the welfare of those involved and those affected.
- **Accuracy:** Evaluation is comprehensive and grounded in the data.

> It is critical to remember that these standards apply to *all* steps and phases of the evaluation plan.

(The Joint Committee on Standards for Educational Evaluation, 1994)

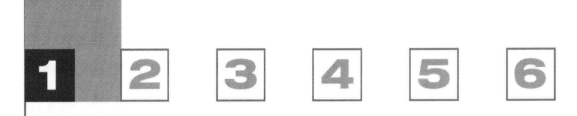

## THE PROCESS OF PARTICIPATORY EVALUATION PLANNING

### Step 1: Engage Stakeholders

#### Defining the Purpose in the Plan

Identifying the purpose of the evaluation is equally as important as identifying the end users or stakeholders who will be part of a consultative group. These two aspects of the evaluation serve as a foundation for evaluation planning, focus, design, and interpretation and use of results. The purpose of an evaluation influences the identification of stakeholders for the evaluation, selection of specific evaluation questions, and the timing of evaluation activities. It is critical that the program is transparent about intended purposes of the evaluation. If evaluation results will be used to determine whether a program should be continued or eliminated, stakeholders should know this up front. The stated purpose of the evaluation drives the expectations and sets the boundaries for what the evaluation can and cannot deliver. In any single evaluation, and especially in a multi-year plan, more than one purpose may be identified; however, the primary purpose can influence resource allocation, use, stakeholders included, and more. Purpose priorities in the plan can help establish the link between purposes and intended use of evaluation information. While there are many ways of stating the identified purpose(s) of the evaluation, they generally fall into three primary categories:

1. Rendering judgments—accountability

2. Facilitating improvements—program development

3. Knowledge generation—transferability

(Patton, 2008)

An ***Evaluation Purpose*** *identification tool/worksheet is provided in Part II, Section 1.2 to assist you with determining intended purposes for your evaluation.*

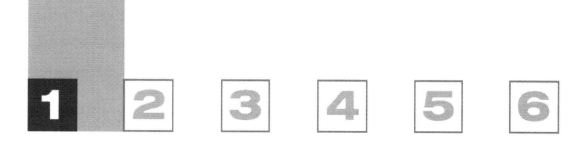

## The ESW: Why should you engage stakeholders in developing the evaluation plan?

A primary feature of an evaluation plan is the identification of an ESW, which includes members who have a stake or vested interest in the evaluation findings, those who are the intended users who can most directly benefit from the evaluation (Patton, 2008; Knowlton, Philips, 2009), as well as others who have a direct or indirect interest in program implementation. Engaging stakeholders in the ESW enhances intended users' understanding and acceptance of the utility of evaluation information. Stakeholders are much more likely to buy into and support the evaluation if they are involved in the evaluation process from the beginning. Moreover, to ensure that the information collected, analyzed, and reported successfully meets the needs of the program and stakeholders, it is best to work with the people who will be using this information throughout the entire process.

---

A **Stakeholder Information Needs** identification exercise is provided in Part II, Section 1.4 to assist you with determining stakeholder information needs.

---

Engaging stakeholders in an evaluation can have many benefits. In general, stakeholders include people who will use the evaluation results, support or maintain the program, or who are affected by the program activities or evaluation results. Stakeholders can help—

- determine and prioritize key evaluation questions,
- pretest data collection instruments,
- facilitate data collection,
- implement evaluation activities,
- increase credibility of analysis and interpretation of evaluation information, and
- ensure evaluation results are used.

*The ESW is comprised of members who have a stake or vested interest in the evaluation findings and can most directly benefit from the evaluation. These members represent the primary users of the evaluation results and generally act as a consultative group throughout the entire planning process, as well as the implementation of the evaluation. Additionally, members sometimes facilitate the implementation and/or the dissemination of results. Examples include promoting responses to surveys, in-kind support for interviews, and interpretation meetings. The members can even identify resources to support evaluation efforts. The exact nature and roles of group members is up to you, but roles should be explicitly delineated and agreed to in the evaluation plan.*

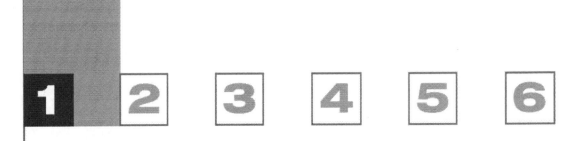

Several questions pertaining to stakeholders may arise among program staff, including:

- Who are the program's stakeholders?
- How can we work with *all* of our stakeholders?
- How are stakeholders' role(s) described in the plan?

This section will help programs address these and other questions about stakeholders and their roles in the evaluation to guide them in writing an effective evaluation plan.

## Who are the program's stakeholders?

The first question to answer when the program begins to write its evaluation plan is to decide which stakeholders to include. Stakeholders are consumers of the evaluation results. As consumers, they will have a vested interest in the results of the evaluation. In general, stakeholders are those who are 1) interested in the program and would use evaluation results, such as clients, community groups, and elected officials; 2) those who are involved in running the program, such as program staff, partners, management, the funding source, and coalition members; and 3) those who are served by the program, their families, or the general public. Others may also be included as these categories are not exclusive.

## How do you use an ESW to develop an evaluation plan?

It is often said of public health programs, "everyone is your stakeholder." Stakeholders will often have diverse and, at times, competing interests. Given that a single evaluation cannot answer all possible evaluation questions raised by diverse groups it will be critical that the prioritization process is outlined in the evaluation plan and that the stakeholder groups represented are identified.

It is suggested that the program enlist the aid of an ESW of 8 to 10 members that represents the stakeholders who have the greatest stake or vested interest in the evaluation (Centers for Disease Control, 2008). These stakeholders, or primary intended users, will serve in a consultative role on all phases of the evaluation. As members of the ESW, they will be an integral part of the entire evaluation process from the initial design phase to interpretation, dissemination, and ensuring use. Stakeholders will play a major role in the program's evaluation, including consultation and possibly even data collection, interpretation, and decision making based on the evaluation results. Sometimes stakeholders can have competing interests that may come to light in the evaluation planning process. It is important to explore agendas in the beginning and come to a shared

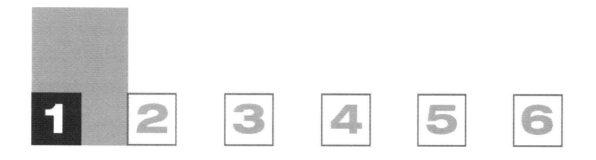

understanding of roles and responsibilities, as well as the purposes of the evaluation. It is important that both the program and the ESW understand and agree to the importance and role of the workgroup in this process.

In order to meaningfully engage your stakeholders, you will need to allow time for resolving conflicts and coming to a shared understanding of the program and evaluation. However, the time is worth the effort and leads toward a truly participatory, empowerment approach to evaluation.

## How are stakeholder's roles described in the plan?

It is important to document information within your written evaluation plan based on the context of your program. For the ESW to be truly integrated into the process, ideally, they will be identified in the evaluation plan. The form this takes may vary based on program needs. If it is important politically, a program might want to specifically name each member of the workgroup, their affiliation, and specific role(s) on the workgroup. If a workgroup is designed with rotating membership by group, then the program might just list the groups represented. For example, a program might have a workgroup that is comprised of members that represent funded programs (three members), non-funded programs (one member), and national partners (four members) or a workgroup that is comprised of members that represent state programs (two members), community programs (five members), and external evaluation expertise (two members). Being transparent about the role and purpose of the ESW can facilitate buy-in for evaluation results from those who did not participate in the evaluation—especially in situations where the evaluation is implemented by internal staff members. Another by-product of workgroup membership is that stakeholders and partners increase their capacity for evaluation activities and increase their ability to be savvy consumers of evaluation information. This can have downstream impacts on stakeholder's and partner's programs such as program improvement and timely, informed decision making. A stakeholder inclusion chart or table can be a useful tool to include in your evaluation plan.

*A **Stakeholder Mapping** exercise and engagement tool/worksheet is provided in Part II, Sections 1.1 and 1.1b to assist you with planning for your evaluation workgroup.*

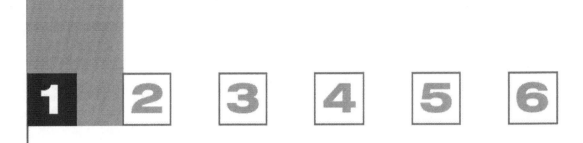

The process for stakeholder engagement should also be described in other steps related to the development of the evaluation plan, which may include:

**Step 2: Describe the program.** A shared understanding of the program and what the evaluation can and cannot deliver is essential to the success of implementation of evaluation activities and use of evaluation results. The program and stakeholders must agree upon the logic model, stage of development description, and purpose(s) of the evaluation.

**Step 3: Focus the evaluation.** Understanding the purpose of the evaluation and the rationale for prioritization of evaluation questions is critical for transparency and acceptance of evaluation findings. It is essential that the evaluation address those questions of greatest need to the program and priority users of the evaluation.

**Step 4: Planning for gathering credible evidence.** Stakeholders have to accept that the methods selected are appropriate to the questions asked and that the data collected are credible or the evaluation results will not be accepted or used. The market for and acceptance of evaluation results begins in the planning phase. Stakeholders can inform the selection of appropriate methods.

**Step 5: Planning for conclusions.** Stakeholders should inform the analysis and interpretation of findings and facilitate the development of conclusions and recommendations. This in turn will facilitate the acceptance and use of the evaluation results by other stakeholder groups. Stakeholders can help determine if and when stakeholder interpretation meetings should be conducted.

**Step 6: Planning for dissemination and sharing of lessons learned.** Stakeholders should inform the translation of evaluation results into practical applications and actively participate in the meaningful dissemination of lessons learned. This will facilitate ensuring use of the evaluation. Stakeholders can facilitate the development of an intentional, strategic communication and dissemination plan within the evaluation plan.

**1** 2 3 4 5 6

EVALUATION PLAN TIPS FOR STEP 1

- Identify intended users who can directly benefit from and use the evaluation results.
- Identify a evaluation stakeholder workgroup of 8 to 10 members.
- Engage stakeholders throughout the plan development process as well as the implementation of the evaluation.
- Identify intended purposes of the evaluation.
- Allow for adequate time to meaningfully engage the evaluation stakeholder workgroup.

EVALUATION TOOLS AND RESOURCES FOR STEP 1:

- 1.1 Stakeholder Mapping Exercise
- 1.1b Stakeholder Mapping Exercise Example
- 1.2 Evaluation Purpose Exercise
- 1.3 Stakeholder Inclusion and Communication Plan Exercise
- 1.4 Stakeholder Information Needs

*AT THIS POINT IN YOUR PLAN, YOU HAVE—*

- *identified the primary users of the evaluation,*
- *created the evaluation stakeholder workgroup, and*
- *defined the purposes of the evaluation.*

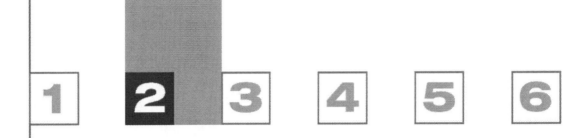

## Step 2: Describe the Program

### Shared Understanding of the Program

The next step in the CDC Framework and the evaluation plan is to describe the program. A program description clarifies the program's purpose, stage of development, activities, capacity to improve health, and implementation context. A shared understanding of the program and what the evaluation can and cannot deliver is essential to the successful implementation of evaluation activities and use of evaluation results. The program and stakeholders must agree upon the logic model, stage of development description, and purpose(s) of the evaluation. This work will set the stage for identifying the program evaluation questions, focusing the evaluation design, and connecting program planning and evaluation.

> A program description clarifies the program's purpose, stage of development, activities, capacity to improve health, and implementation context.

### Narrative Description

A narrative description helps ensure a full and complete shared understanding of the program. A logic model may be used to succinctly synthesize the main elements of a program. While a logic model is not always necessary, a program narrative is. The program description is essential for focusing the evaluation design and selecting the appropriate methods. Too often groups jump to evaluation methods before they even have a grasp of what the program is designed to achieve or what the evaluation should deliver. Even though much of this will have been included in your funding application, it is good practice to revisit this description with your ESW to ensure a shared understanding and that the program is still being implemented as intended. The description will be based on your program's objectives and context but most descriptions include at a minimum:

- **A statement of need** to identify the health issue addressed
- **Inputs or program resources** available to implement program activities
- **Program activities** linked to program outcomes through theory or best practice program logic
- **Stage of development** of the program to reflect program maturity
- **Environmental context** within which a program is implemented

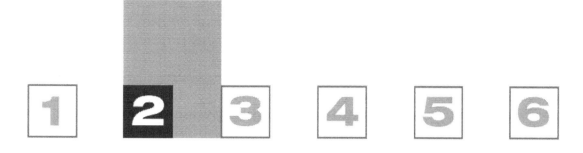

## Logic Model

The description section often includes a logic model to visually show the link between activities and intended outcomes. It is helpful to review the model with the ESW to ensure a shared understanding of the model and that the logic model is still an accurate and complete reflection of your program. The logic model should identify available resources (inputs), what the program is doing (activities), and what you hope to achieve (outcomes). You might also want to articulate any challenges you face (the program's context or environment). Figure 2 illustrates the basic components of a program logic model. As you view the logic model from left to right, the further away from the intervention the more time needed to observe outcomes. A major challenge in evaluating chronic disease prevention and health promotion programs is one of attribution versus contribution and the fact that distal outcomes may not occur in close proximity to the program interventions or policy change. In addition, given the complexities of dynamic implementation environments, realized impacts may differ from intended impacts. However, the rewards of understanding the proximal and distal impacts of the program intervention often outweigh the challenges.

Logic model elements include:

**Inputs:** Resources necessary for program implementation

**Activities:** The actual interventions that the program implements in order to achieve health outcomes

**Outputs:** Direct products obtained as a result of program activities

**Outcomes** (short-term, intermediate, long-term, distal): The changes, impacts, or results of program implementation (activities and outputs)

Figure 2: Sample Logic Model

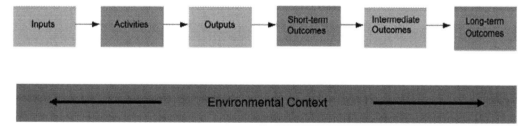

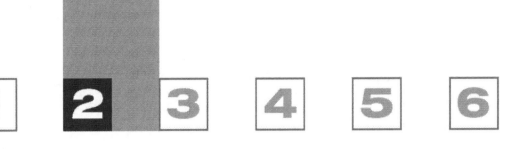

## Stage of Development

Another activity that will be needed to fully describe your program and prepare you to focus your evaluation is an accurate assessment of the stage of development of the program. The developmental stages that programs typically move through are **planning, implementation, and maintenance**. In the example of a policy or environmental initiative, the stages might look somewhat like this:

1. Assess environment and assets.
2. Policy or environmental change is in development.
3. The policy or environmental change has not yet been approved.
4. The policy or environmental change has been approved but not implemented.
5. The policy or environmental change has been in effect for less than 1 year.
6. The policy or environmental change has been in effect for 1 year or longer.

Steps 1 through 3 would typically fall under the planning stages, Steps 4 and 5 under implementation, and Step 6 under maintenance. It is important to consider a developmental model because programs are dynamic and evolve over time. Programs are seldom fixed in stone and progress is affected by many aspects of the political and economic context. When it comes to evaluation, the stages are not always a "once-and-done" sequence of events. When a program has progressed past the initial planning stage, it may experience occasions where environment and asset assessment is still needed. Additionally, in a multi-year plan, the evaluation should consider future evaluation plans to prepare datasets and baseline information for evaluation projects considering more distal impacts and outcomes. This is an advantage of completing a multi-year evaluation plan with your ESW—preparation!

The stage of development conceptual model is complementary to the logic model. Figure 3.1 shows how general program evaluation questions are distinguished by both logic model categories and the developmental stage of the program. This places evaluation within the appropriate stage of program development (planning, implementation, and maintenance). The model offers suggested starting points for asking evaluation questions within the logic model while respecting the developmental stage of the program. This will prepare the program and the workgroup to focus the evaluation appropriately based on program maturity and priorities.

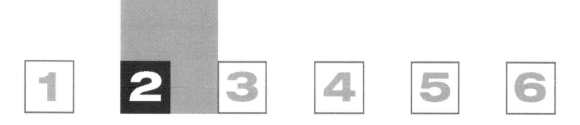

Figure 3.1: Stage of Development by Logic Model Category

| Developmental Stage | Program Planning | Program Implementation | Program Maintenance |
|---|---|---|---|
| Logic Model Category | Inputs and Activities | Outputs and Short-term Outcomes | Intermediate and Long-term Outcomes |

Figure 3.2: Stage of Development by Logic Model Category Example

| Developmental Stage | Program Planning | Program Implementation | Program Maintenance |
|---|---|---|---|
| Example: Developmental Stages When Passing a Policy | Assess environment and assets<br><br>Develop policy<br><br>The policy has not yet been passed | The policy has been passed but not implemented<br><br>The policy has been in effect for less than 1 year | The policy has been in effect for 1 year or longer |
| Example: Questions Based on Developmental Stage When Passing a Policy | Is there public support for the policy?<br><br>What resources will be needed for implementation of the policy? | Is there compliance with the policy?<br><br>Is there continued or increased public support for the policy?<br><br>Are there major exemptions or loopholes to the policy? | What is the health impact of the policy? |

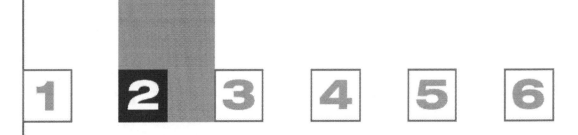

Key evaluation questions and needs for information will differ based on the stage of development of the program. Additionally, the ability to answer key evaluation questions will differ by stage of development of the program and stakeholders need to be aware of what the evaluation can and cannot answer. For the above policy program example, planning stage type questions might include:

- Is there public support for the policy?
- What resources will be needed for implementation of the policy?

Implementation stage questions might include:

- Is there compliance with the policy?
- Is there continued or increased public support for the policy?
- Are there major exemptions or loopholes to the policy?

Maintenance stage questions might include:

- What is the economic impact of the policy?
- What is the health impact of the policy?

For more on stage of development and Smoke-Free Policies, please see the Evaluation Toolkit for Smoke-Free Policies at http://www.cdc.gov/tobacco/basic_information/secondhand_smoke/evaluation_toolkit/index.htm.

---

*A **Program Stage of Development** exercise is included in Part II, Section 2.1.*

---

EVALUATION PLAN TIPS FOR STEP 2

- A program description will facilitate a shared understanding of the program between the program staff and the evaluation workgroup.
- The description section often includes a logic model to visually show the link between activities and intended outcomes.
- The logic model should identify available resources (inputs), what the program is doing (activities), and what you hope to achieve (outcomes).
- A quality program evaluation is most effective when part of a larger conceptual model of a program and its development.

EVALUATION TOOLS AND RESOURCES FOR STEP 2:

- 2.1 Program Stage of Development Exercise
- Evaluation Toolkit for Smoke-Free Policies at http://www.cdc.gov/tobacco/ basic_information/secondhand_smoke/evaluation_toolkit/index.htm

*AT THIS POINT IN YOUR PLAN, YOU HAVE—*

*identified the primary users of the evaluation,*
*created the evaluation stakeholder workgroup,*
*defined the purposes of the evaluation,*
*described the program, including context,*
*created a shared understanding of the program, and*
*identified the stage of development of the program.*

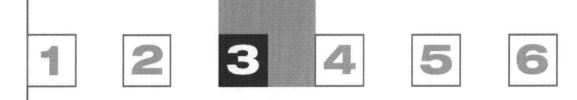

## Step 3: Focus the Evaluation

The amount of information you can gather concerning your program is potentially limitless. Evaluations, however, are always restricted by the number of questions that can be realistically asked and answered with quality, the methods that can be employed, the feasibility of data collection, and the available resources. These are the issues at the heart of Step 3 in the CDC framework: focusing the evaluation. The scope and depth of any program evaluation is dependent on program and stakeholder priorities; available resources, including financial resources; staff and contractor availability; and amount of time committed to the evaluation. The program staff should work together with the ESW to determine the priority and feasibility of these questions and identify the uses of results before designing the evaluation plan. In this part of the plan, you will apply the purposes of the evaluation, its uses, and the program description to narrow the evaluation questions and focus the evaluation for program improvement and decision making. In this step, you may begin to notice the iterative process of developing the evaluation plan as you revisit aspects of Step 1 and Step 2 to inform decisions to be made in Step 3.

Useful evaluations are not about special research interests or what is easiest to implement but what information *will be used* by the program, stakeholders (including funders), and decision makers to improve the program and make decisions. Establishing the focus of the evaluation began with the identification of the primary purposes and the primary intended users of the evaluation. This process was further solidified through the selection of the ESW. Developing the purposeful intention to *use* evaluation information and not just produce another evaluation report starts at the very beginning with program planning and your evaluation plan. You need to garner stakeholder interests and prepare them for evaluation use. This step facilitates conceptualizing what the evaluation can and cannot deliver.

It is important to collaboratively focus the evaluation design with your ESW based on the identified purposes, program context, logic model, and stage of development. Additionally, issues of priority, feasibility, and efficiency need to be discussed with the ESW and those responsible for the implementation of the evaluation. Transparency is particularly important in this step. Stakeholders and users of the evaluation will need to understand why some questions were identified as high priorities while others were rejected or delayed.

*A **Focus the Evaluation** exercise is located in Part II, Section 3.1 of this workbook.*

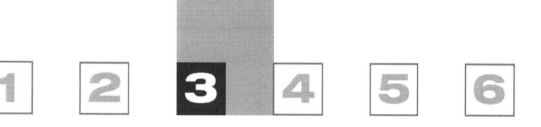

## Developing Evaluation Questions

In this step, it is important to solicit evaluation questions from your various stakeholder groups based on the stated purposes of the evaluation. The questions should then be considered through the lens of the logic model/program description and stage of development of the program. Evaluation questions should be checked against the logic model and changes may be made to either the questions or the logic model, thus reinforcing the iterative nature of the evaluation planning process. The stage of development discussed in the previous chapter will facilitate narrowing the evaluation questions even further. It is important to remember that a program may experience characteristics of several stages simultaneously once past the initial planning stage. You may want to ask yourself this question: *How long has your program been in existence?* If your program is in the planning stage, it is unlikely that measuring distal outcomes will be useful for informing program decision making. However, in a multi-year evaluation plan, you may begin to plan for and develop the appropriate surveillance and evaluation systems and baseline information needed to measure these distal outcomes (to be conducted in the final initiative year) as early as year 1. In another scenario, you may have a coalition that has been established for 10 years and is in maintenance stage. However, contextual changes may require you to rethink the programmatic approach being taken. In this situation, you may want to do an evaluation that looks at both planning stage questions ("Are the right folks at the table?" and "Are they really engaged?"), as well as maintenance stage questions ("Are we having the intended programmatic impact?"). Questions can be further prioritized based on the ESW and program information needs as well as feasibility and efficiency issues.

Often if a funder requires an evaluation plan, you might notice text like this:

*Submit with application a comprehensive written evaluation plan that includes activities for both process and outcome measures.*

Distinguishing between process and outcome evaluation can be similar to considering the stage of development of your program against your program logic model. In general, process evaluation focuses on the first three boxes of the logic model: inputs, activities, and outputs (CDC, 2008). This discussion with your ESW can further facilitate the focus of your evaluation.

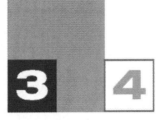

| 1 | 2 | **3** | 4 | 5 | 6 |

**Process and Outcome Evaluation in Harmony in the Evaluation Plan**

*As the program can experience the characteristics of several stages of development at once, so, too, a single evaluation plan can and often does include both process and outcome evaluation questions. Excluding process evaluation questions in favor of outcome evaluation questions often eliminates the understanding of the foundation that supports outcomes. Additional resources on process and outcome evaluation are identified in the Resource Section of this workbook.*

Process Evaluation Focus

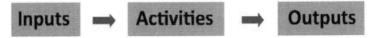

Process evaluation enables you to describe and assess your program's activities and to link your progress to outcomes. This is important because the link between outputs and short-term outcomes remains an empirical question.

(CDC, 2008)

Outcome evaluation, as the term implies, focuses on the last three outcome boxes of the logic model: short-term, intermediate, and long-term outcomes.

Outcome Evaluation Focus

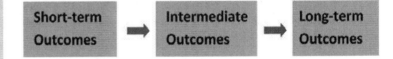

Outcome evaluation allows researchers to document health and behavioral outcomes and identify linkages between an intervention and quantifiable effects.

(CDC, 2008)

As a program can experience the characteristics of several stages of development at once, so, too, a single evaluation plan can and should include both process and outcome evaluation questions at the same time. Excluding process evaluation questions in favor of outcome evaluation questions often eliminates the understanding of the foundation that supports outcomes.

As you and the ESW take ownership of the evaluation, you will find that honing the evaluation focus will likely solidify interest in the evaluation. Selection of final evaluation questions should balance what is most useful to achieving your program's information needs while also meeting your stakeholders' information needs. Having stakeholders participate in the selection of questions increases the likelihood of their securing evaluation

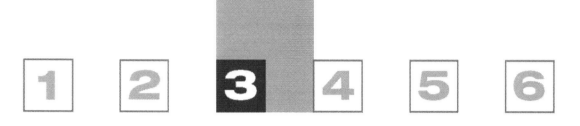

resources, providing access to data, and using the results. This process increases "personal ownership" of the evaluation by the ESW. However, given that resources are limited, the evaluation cannot answer all potential questions.

The ultimate goal is to focus the evaluation design such that it reflects the program stage of development, selected purpose of the evaluation, uses, and questions to be answered. Transparency related to the selection of evaluation questions is critical to stakeholder acceptance of evaluation results and possibly even for continued support of the program.

Even with an established multi-year plan, Step 3 should be revisited with your ESW annually (or more often if needed) to determine if priorities and feasibility issues still hold for the planned evaluation activities. This highlights the dynamic nature of the evaluation plan. Ideally, your plan should be intentional and strategic by design and generally cover multiple years for planning purposes. But the plan is not set in stone. It should also be flexible and adaptive. It is flexible because resources and priorities change and adaptive because opportunities and programs change. You may have a new funding opportunity and a short-term program added to your overall program. This may require insertion of a smaller evaluation plan specific to the newly funded project, but with the overall program evaluation goals and objectives in mind. Or, resources could be cut for a particular program requiring a reduction in the evaluation budget. The planned evaluation may have to be reduced or delayed. Your evaluation plan should be flexible and adaptive to accommodate these scenarios while still focusing on the evaluation goals and objectives of the program and the ESW.

## Budget and Resources

Discussion of budget and resources (financial and human) that can be allocated to the evaluation will likely be included in your feasibility discussion. In the Best Practices for Comprehensive Tobacco Control Programs (2007), it is recommended that at least 10% of your total program resources be allocated to surveillance and program evaluation. The questions and subsequent methods selected will have a direct relationship to the financial resources available, evaluation team member skills, and environmental constraints (e.g., you might like to do an in-person home interview of the target population, but the neighborhood is not one that interviewers can visit safely). Stakeholder involvement may facilitate advocating for the resources needed to implement the evaluation necessary to answer priority questions. However, sometimes, you might not have the resources necessary to fund the evaluation questions you would like to answer most. A thorough

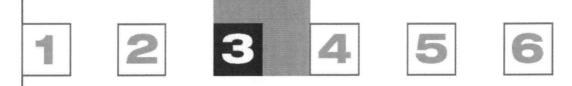

discussion of feasibility and recognition of real constraints will facilitate a shared understanding of what the evaluation can and cannot deliver. The process of selecting the appropriate methods to answer the priority questions and discussing feasibility and efficiency is iterative. Steps 3, 4, and 5 in planning the evaluation will often be visited concurrently in a back-and-forth progression until the group comes to consensus.

---

**EVALUATION PLAN TIPS FOR STEP 3**

- It is not possible or appropriate to evaluate every aspect or specific initiative of a program every year.
- Evaluation focus is context dependent and related to the purposes of the evaluation, primary users, stage of development, logic model, program priorities, and feasibility.
- Evaluation questions should be checked against the logic model and stage of development of the program.
- The iterative nature of plan development is reinforced in this step.

**EVALUATION TOOLS AND RESOURCES FOR STEP 3:**

- 3.1 Focus the Evaluation Exercise

---

*AT THIS POINT IN YOUR PLAN, YOU HAVE—*

- *identified the primary users of the evaluation,*
- *created the evaluation stakeholder workgroup,*
- *defined the purposes of the evaluation,*
- *described the program, including context,*
- *created a shared understanding of the program,*
- *identified the stage of development of the program, and*
- *prioritized evaluation questions and discussed feasibility, budget, and resource issues.*

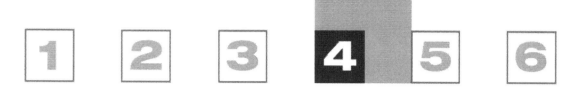

## Step 4: Planning for Gathering Credible Evidence

Now that you have solidified the focus of your evaluation and identified the questions to be answered, it will be necessary to select the *appropriate methods that fit the evaluation questions you have selected*. Sometimes the approach to evaluation planning is guided by a favorite method(s) and the evaluation is forced to fit that method. This could lead to incomplete or inaccurate answers to evaluation questions.

Ideally, the evaluation questions inform the methods. If you have followed the steps in the workbook, you have collaboratively chosen the evaluation questions with your ESW that will provide you with information that will be used for program improvement and decision making. This is documented and transparent in your evaluation plan. *Now is the time to select the most appropriate method to fit the evaluation questions and describe the selection process in your plan*. Additionally, it is prudent to identify in your plan a timeline and the roles and responsibilities of those overseeing the evaluation activity implementation whether it is program or stakeholder staff.

To accomplish this step in your evaluation plan, you will need to—

- keep in mind the purpose, logic model/program description, stage of development of the program, evaluation questions, and what the evaluation can and cannot deliver,
- confirm that the method(s) fits the question(s); there are a multitude of options, including but not limited to qualitative, quantitative, mixed-methods, multiple methods, naturalistic inquiry, experimental, quasi-experimental,
- think about what will constitute credible evidence for stakeholders or users,
- identify sources of evidence (e.g., persons, documents, observations, administrative databases, surveillance systems) and appropriate methods for obtaining quality (i.e., reliable and valid) data,
- identify roles and responsibilities along with timelines to ensure the project remains on-time and on-track, and
- remain flexible and adaptive, and as always, transparent.

> ***Fitting the Method to the Evaluation Question(s)***
>
> *The method or methods chosen need to fit the evaluation question(s) and not be chosen just because they are a favored method or specifically quantitative or experimental in nature. A misfit between evaluation question and method can and often does lead to incomplete or even inaccurate information. The method needs to be appropriate for the question in accordance with the Evaluation Standards.*

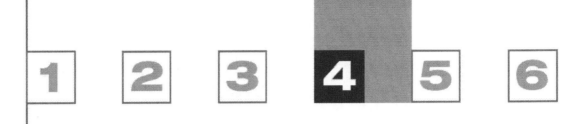

## Choosing the Appropriate Methods

It is at this point that the debate between qualitative and quantitative methods usually arises. It is not that one method is right and one method is wrong, but which method or combination of methods will obtain answers to the evaluation questions.

Some options that may point you in the direction of qualitative methods:

- You are planning and want to assess what to consider when designing a program or initiative. You want to identify elements that are likely to be effective.
- You are looking for feedback while a program or initiative is in its early stages and want to implement a process evaluation. You want to understand approaches to enhance the likelihood that an initiative (e.g., policy or environmental change) will be adopted.
- Something isn't working as expected and you need to know why. You need to understand the facilitators and barriers to implementation of a particular initiative.
- You want to truly understand how a program is implemented on the ground and need to develop a model or theory of the program or initiative.

Some options that may point you in the direction of quantitative methods:

- You are looking to identify current and future movement or trends of a particular phenomenon or initiative.
- You want to consider standardized outcome across programs. You need to monitor outputs and outcomes of an initiative. You want to document the impact of a particular initiative.
- You want to know the costs associated with the implementation of a particular intervention.
- You want to understand what standardized outcomes are connected with a particular initiative and need to develop a model or theory of the program or initiative.

Or the most appropriate method may be a mixed methods approach wherein the qualitative data provide value, understanding, and application to the quantitative data. It is beyond the scope of this workbook to address the full process of deciding what method(s) are most appropriate for which types of evaluations questions. The question is not whether to apply qualitative or quantitative methods but what method is most appropriate to answer the evaluation question chosen. Additional resources on this are provided in the resource section in Part II.

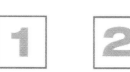  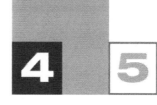 

## Credible Evidence

The evidence you gather to support the answers to your evaluation questions should be seen as credible by the primary users of the evaluation. The determination of what is credible is often context dependent and can vary across programs and stakeholders. This determination is naturally tied to the evaluation design, implementation, and standards adhered to for data collection, analysis, and interpretation. Best practices for your program area and the evaluation standards included in the CDC Framework (Utility, Feasibility, Propriety, and Accuracy) and espoused by the

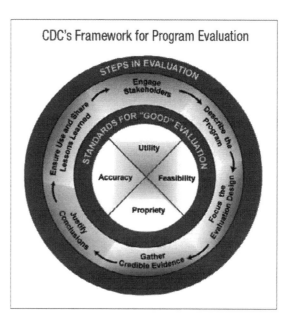

CDC's Framework for Program Evaluation

American Evaluation Association (http://www.eval.org) will facilitate this discussion with your ESW. This discussion allows for stakeholder input as to what methods are most appropriate given the questions and context of your evaluation. As with all the steps, transparency is important to the credibility discussion as well as the documentation of limitation of the evaluation methods or design. This facilitates the likelihood that results will be more acceptable to stakeholders and strengthens the value of the evaluation and likelihood the information will be used for program improvement and decision making. The value of stakeholder inclusion throughout the development of your evaluation plan is prominent in Step 4. More information on the standards can be found in the resources section.

## Measurement

If the method selected includes indicators and/or performance measures, the discussion of what measures to include is critical and often lengthy. This discussion is naturally tied to the data credibility conversation, and there is often a wide range of possible indicators or performance measures that can be selected for any one evaluation question. You will want to consult best practices publications for your program area and even other programs in neighboring states or locales. The expertise that your ESW brings to the table can facilitate this discussion. The exact selection of indicators or performance measures is beyond the scope of this workbook. Resource information is included in Part II of this workbook, such as the *Key Outcome Indicators for Evaluating Comprehensive Tobacco Programs* guide.

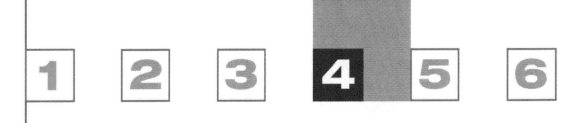

## Data Sources and Methods

As emphasized already, it is important to select the method(s) *most appropriate to answer the evaluation question*. The types of data needed should be reviewed and considered for credibility and feasibility. Based on the methods chosen, you may need a variety of input, such as case studies, interviews, naturalistic inquiry, focus groups, standardized indicators, and surveys. You may need to consider multiple data sources and the triangulation of data for reliability and validity of your information. Data may come from existing sources (e.g., Behavioral Risk Factor Surveillance System, Youth Risk Behavior Surveillance, Pregnancy Risk Assessment Monitoring System) or gathered from program-specific sources (either existing or new). You most likely will need to consider the establishment of surveillance and evaluation systems for continuity and the ability to successfully conduct useful evaluations. The form of the data (either quantitative or qualitative) and specifics of how these data will be collected must be defined, agreed upon as credible, and transparent. There are strengths and limitations to any approach, and they should be considered carefully with the help of your ESW. For example, the use of existing data sources may help reduce costs, maximize the use of existing information, and facilitate comparability with other programs, but may not provide program specificity. Additionally, existing sources of data may not meet the question-method appropriateness criteria.

It is beyond the scope of this workbook to discuss in detail the complexities of what appropriate method(s) or data sources to choose. It is important to remember that not all methods fit all evaluation questions and often a mixed-methods approach is the best option for a comprehensive answer to a particular evaluation question. This is often where you need to consult with your evaluation experts for direction on matching method to question. More information can be found through the resources listed in Part II. Note that all data collected needs to have a clear link to the associated evaluation question and anticipated use to reduce unnecessary burden on the respondent and stakeholders. It is important to revisit data collection efforts over the course of a multi-year evaluation plan to examine utility against the burden on respondents and stakeholders. Finally, this word of caution—it is not enough to have defined measures. Quality assurance procedures must be put into place so that data is collected in a reliable way, coded and entered correctly, and checked for accuracy. A quality assurance plan should be included in your evaluation plan.

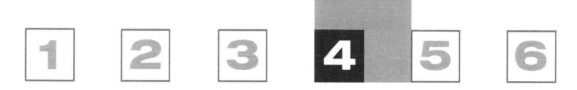

## Roles and Responsibilities

Writing an evaluation plan will not ensure that the evaluation is implemented on time, as intended, or within budget. A critical piece of the evaluation plan is to identify the roles and responsibilities of program staff, evaluation staff, contractors, and stakeholders from the beginning of the planning process. This information should be kept up to date throughout the implementation of the evaluation. Stakeholders must clearly understand their role in the evaluation implementation. Maintaining an involved, engaged network of stakeholders throughout the development and implementation of the plan will increase the likelihood that their participation serves the needs of the evaluation. An evaluation implementation work plan is as critical to the success of the evaluation as a program work plan is to the success of the program. This is even more salient when multiple organizations are involved and/or multiple evaluation activities occur simultaneously.

## Evaluation Plan Methods Grid

One tool that is particularly useful in your evaluation plan is an **evaluation plan methods grid**. Not only is this tool helpful to align evaluation questions with methods, indicators, performance measures, data sources, roles, and responsibilities but it can facilitate a shared understanding of the overall evaluation plan with stakeholders. The tool can take many forms and should be adapted to fit your specific evaluation and context.

Figure 4.1: Evaluation Plan Methods Grid Example

| Evaluation Question | Indicator/ Performance Measure | Method | Data Source | Frequency | Responsibility |
|---|---|---|---|---|---|
| What process leads to implementation of policy? | Interview description of process steps, actions, and strategies | Case study, interviews, document reviews etc. | Site visits and reports | Pre and post funding period | Contractor |

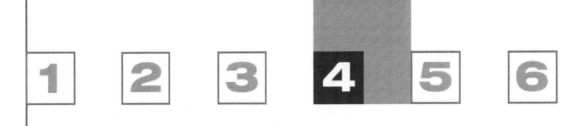

Figure 4.2: Evaluation Plan Methods Grid Example

| Evaluation Question | Indicators/ Performance Measure | Potential Data Source (Existing/New) | Comments |
|---|---|---|---|
| What media promotion activities are being implemented? | Description of promotional activities and their reach of targeted populations, dose, intensity | Focus group feedback<br>Target Rating Point and Gross Rating Point data sources<br>Enrollment data | |

An **Evaluation Plan Methods Grid** exercise and more examples can be found in Part II, Section 4.1.

## Budget

The evaluation budget discussion was most likely initially started during Step 3 when the team was discussing the focus of the evaluation and feasibility issues. It is now time to develop a complete evaluation project budget based on the decisions made about the evaluation questions, methods, roles, and responsibilities of stakeholders. A complete budget is necessary to ensure that the evaluation project is fully funded and can deliver upon promises.

An **Evaluation Budget** exercise and more examples can be found in Part II, Section 4.2.

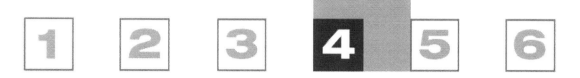

EVALUATION PLAN TIPS FOR STEP 4

- Select the best method(s) that answers the evaluation question. This can often involve a mixed-methods approach.
- Gather the evidence that is seen as credible by the primary users of the evaluation.
- Define implementation roles and responsibilities for program staff, evaluation staff, contractors, and stakeholders.
- Develop an evaluation plan methods grid to facilitate a shared understanding of the overall evaluation plan, and the timeline for evaluation activities.

EVALUATION TOOLS AND RESOURCES FOR STEP 4:

- 4.1 Evaluation Plan Methods Grid Exercise
- 4.2 Evaluation Budget Exercise

*AT THIS POINT IN YOUR PLAN, YOU HAVE—*

- *identified the primary users of the evaluation,*
- *created the evaluation stakeholder workgroup,*
- *defined the purposes of the evaluation,*
- *described the program, including context,*
- *created a shared understanding of the program,*
- *identified the stage of development of the program,*
- *prioritized evaluation questions and discussed feasibility issues,*
- *discussed issues related to credibility of data sources,*
- *identified indicators and/or performance measures linked to chosen evaluation questions,*
- *determined implementation roles and responsibilities for program staff, evaluation staff, contractors, and stakeholders, and*
- *developed an evaluation plan methods grid.*

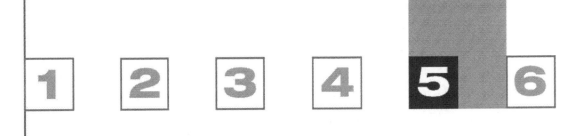

## Step 5: Planning for Conclusions

Justifying conclusions includes analyzing the information you collect, interpreting, and drawing conclusions from your data. This step is needed to turn the data collected into meaningful, useful, and accessible information. This is often when programs incorrectly assume they no longer need the ESW integrally involved in decision making and instead look to the "experts" to complete the analyses and interpretation. However, engaging the ESW in this step is critical to ensuring the meaningfulness, credibility, and acceptance of evaluation findings and conclusions. Actively meeting with stakeholders and discussing preliminary findings helps to guide the interpretation phase. In fact, stakeholders often have novel insights or perspectives to guide interpretation that evaluation staff may not have, leading to more thoughtful conclusions.

Planning for analysis and interpretation is directly tied to the timetable begun in Step 4. Errors or omissions in planning this step can create serious delays in the final evaluation report and may result in missed opportunities if the report has been timed to correspond with significant events. Often, groups fail to appreciate the resources, time, and expertise required to clean and analyze data. This applies to both qualitative and quantitative data. Some programs focus their efforts on collecting data, but never fully appreciate the time it takes to work with the data to prepare for analysis, interpretation, feedback, and conclusions. These programs are suffering from "D.R.I.P.", that is, programs that are "Data Rich but Information Poor." Survey data remains "in boxes" or interviews are never fully explored for theme identification.

After planning for the analysis of the data, you have to prepare to examine the results to determine what the data actually say about your program. These results should be interpreted with the goals of your program in mind, the social/political context of the program, and the needs of the stakeholders.

Moreover, it is critical that your plans include time for interpretation and review by stakeholders to increase transparency and validity of your process and conclusions. The emphasis here is on justifying conclusions, not just analyzing data. This is a step that deserves due diligence in the planning process. The propriety standard plays a role in guiding the evaluator's decisions on how to analyze and interpret data to assure that all stakeholder values are respected in the process of drawing conclusions (Program Evaluation Standards, 1994). That is to say, who needs to be involved in the evaluation for it to be ethical. This may include one or more stakeholder interpretation meetings to review interim data and further refine conclusions. A note of caution, as a stakeholder driven process, there is often pressure to reach beyond the evidence when drawing conclusions.

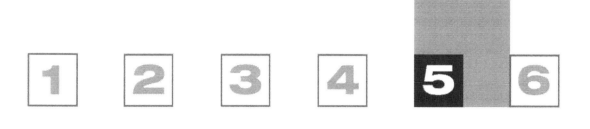

It is the responsibility of the evaluator and the ESW to ensure that conclusions are drawn directly from the evidence. This is a topic that should be discussed with the ESW in the planning stages along with reliability and validity issues and possible sources of biases. If possible and appropriate, triangulation of data should be considered and remedies to threats to the credibility of the data should be addressed as early as possible.

A *Stakeholder Interpretation Meeting* exercise is found in Part II, Section 5.1.

EVALUATION PLAN TIPS FOR STEP 5

- The planning for conclusions step is needed to turn the data collected into meaningful, useful, and accessible information for action.
- Including your stakeholder group in this step is directly tied to the previous discussion on credibility and acceptance of data and conclusions.
- Errors in planning in this step can create serious delays in the final evaluation report and may result in missed opportunities if the report has been timed to correspond to significant events.
- It is critical that your plans include time for interpretation and review from stakeholders (including your critics) to increase transparency and validity of your process and conclusions.

EVALUATION TOOLS AND RESOURCES FOR STEP 5:

- 5.1 Stakeholder Interpretation Meeting Exercise
- Western Michigan University, The Evaluation Center at http://www.wmich.edu/evalctr/checklists/

**AT THIS POINT IN YOUR PLAN, YOU HAVE—**

- *identified the primary users of the evaluation,*
- *created the evaluation stakeholder workgroup,*
- *defined the purposes of the evaluation,*
- *described the program, including context,*
- *created a shared understanding of the program,*
- *identified the stage of development of the program,*
- *prioritized evaluation questions and discussed feasibility issues,*
- *discussed issues related to credibility of data sources,*
- *identified indicators and/or performance measures linked to chosen evaluation questions,*
- *determined implementation roles and responsibilities for program staff, evaluation staff, contractors, and stakeholders,*
- *developed an evaluation plan methods grid,*
- *addressed possible threats to the credibility of your data, and*
- *developed a timetable that includes cleaning and analyzing data as well as stakeholder interpretation sessions.*

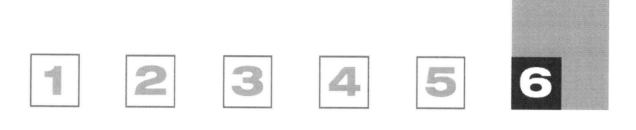

## Step 6: Planning for Dissemination and Sharing of Lessons Learned

Another often overlooked step in the planning stage is Step 6, planning for use of evaluation results, sharing of lessons learned, communication, and dissemination of results. It is often felt that this step will just take care of itself once the report is published. In reality, planning for use begins with Step 1 and the consideration of stakeholder involvement. Evaluation use is likely when end use is planned for and built into the six steps in your evaluation plan. Planning for use is directly tied to the identified purposes of the evaluation and program and stakeholder priorities. Your decision to include the ESW throughout the plan development stage begins the process of building a market for your evaluation results and increases the chances that results will be used for program improvement and decision making. Use of evaluation is most likely to occur when evaluation is collaborative and participatory, a process that begins in the planning phase. This step is directly tied to the utility standard in evaluation. Is it ethical to consume program and stakeholder resources if evaluation results are never used? The resources expended and the information gained from evaluations are too important to just hope that evaluation results will be used. Use must be planned for, nurtured, and included in the evaluation plan from the very beginning.

> Use must be planned for, cultivated, and included in the evaluation plan from the very beginning

Based on the uses for your evaluation, you will need to determine who should learn about the findings and how they should learn the information. Typically, this is where the final report is published, and most assume the evaluation is done. However, if personal ownership of evaluation results is inserted here, such as through collaboration with an ESW, the impact and value of the evaluation results will increase (Patton, 2008). The program and the ESW take personal responsibility for getting the results to the right people and in a usable, targeted format. This absolutely must be planned for and included in the evaluation plan. It will be important to consider the audience in terms of timing, style, tone, message source, method and format. Remember that stakeholders will not suddenly become interested in your product just because you produced a report. You must sufficiently prepare the market for the product and for use of the evaluation results (Patton, 2008). Writing a straightforward and comprehensive evaluation report can help insure use.

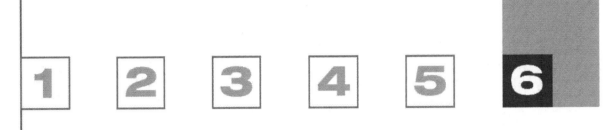

## Communication and Dissemination Plans

Your evaluation results may not reach the intended audience with the intended impact just because they are published. An intentional communication and dissemination approach should be included in your evaluation plan. As previously stated, the planning stage is the time for the program and the ESW to begin to think about the best way to share the lessons you will learn from the evaluation. The communication-dissemination phase of the evaluation is a two-way process designed to support use of the evaluation results for program improvement and decision making. In order to achieve this outcome, a program must translate evaluation results into practical applications and must systematically distribute the information through a variety of audience-specific strategies. In order to be effective, dissemination systems need to—

- orient toward the needs of the user, incorporating the types and levels of information needed into the forms and language preferred by the user,
- use varied dissemination methods, including written information, electronic media, and person-to-person contact,
- include both proactive and reactive dissemination channels—that is, incorporate information that users have identified as important and information that users may not know to request but that they are likely to need,
- establish clear channels for users to make their needs and priorities known to the disseminating agency,
- recognize and provide for the "natural flow" of the four levels of dissemination that have been identified as leading to utilization: spread, exchange, choice, and implementation,
- draw upon existing resources, relationships, and networks to the maximum extent possible while building new resources as needed by users,
- include effective quality control mechanisms to assure that information included is accurate, relevant, and representative,
- incorporate sufficient information so that the user can determine the basic principles underlying specific practices and the settings in which these practices may be used most productively, and
- establish linkages to resources that may be needed to implement the information— usually referred to as technical assistance.

(National Institute on Disability and Rehabilitation Research, 2001)

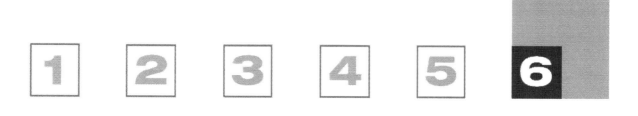

The first step in writing an effective communications plan is to define your communication goals and objectives. Given that the communication objectives will be tailored to each target audience, you need to consider with your ESW who the primary audience(s) are (e.g., the funding agency, the general public, or some other group). Some questions to ask about the potential audience(s) are the following:

- Who is a priority?
- What do they already know about the topic?
- What is critical for them to know?
- Where do they prefer to receive their information?
- What is their preferred format?
- What language level is appropriate?
- Within what time frame are evaluation updates and reports necessary?

Once the goals, objectives, and target audiences of the communication plan are established, you should consider the best way to reach the intended audience by considering which communication/dissemination tools will best serve your goals and objectives. Will the program use newsletters/fact sheets, oral presentations, visual displays, videos, storytelling, and/or press releases? Carefully consider the best tools to use by getting feedback from your ESW, by learning from others' experiences, and by reaching out to target audiences to gather their preferences. An excellent resource to facilitate creative techniques for reporting evaluation results is Torres, Preskill, and Pionteck's (2004) *Evaluation Strategies for Communicating and Reporting.*

Complete the communication planning step by establishing a timetable for sharing evaluation findings and lessons learned. Figure 5 can be useful in helping the program to chart the written communications plan:

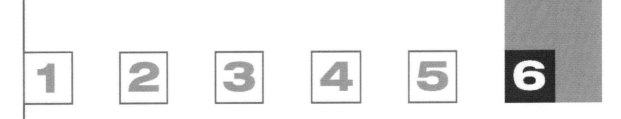

Figure 5: Communication Plan Table

| Target Audience (Priority) | Goals | Tools | Timetable |
|---|---|---|---|
| Program Implementation Team | Inform them in real time about what's working well and what needs to be quickly adjusted during implementation | Monthly meetings and briefing documents | Monthly |
| Program Stakeholders | Promote program progress | Success stories | Annually |
| Funding Decision Makers | Continue and/or enhance program funding | Executive summary; Targeted program briefs | Within 90 days of conclusion of funding |

It is important to note that you do not have to wait until the final evaluation report is written in order to share your evaluation results. A system for sharing interim results to facilitate program course corrections and decision making should be included in your evaluation plan. Additionally, success stories that focus on upstream, midstream, and downstream successes can facilitate program growth and visibility. A success story can show movement in your program's progress over time and demonstrate its value and impact. It can serve as a vehicle for engaging potential participants, partners, and funders especially when it takes time for a program to mature to long-term outcomes (Lavinghouze, Price, Smith, 2007).

The **Communicating Results** exercise can be found in Part II, Section 6.2 and can assist you with tracking your audiences and ways to reach them. More information on developing a communication and dissemination plan can be found in the Resource Section in Part II of this workbook.

1 2 3 4 5 6

## Ensuring Use

Communicating results is not enough to *ensure use* of evaluation results and lessons learned. The evaluation team and program staff needs to proactively take action to encourage use and wide dissemination of the information gleaned through the evaluation project. It is helpful to strategize with stakeholders early in the evaluation process about how your program will ensure that findings are used to support program improvement efforts and inform decision making. Program staff and the ESW must take personal responsibility for guaranteeing the dissemination of and application of evaluation results.

There are several practical steps you can include in your evaluation plan to help ensure evaluation findings are used. These steps might contain plans to—

- conduct regularly scheduled meetings with evaluation stakeholders as a forum for sharing evaluation findings in real time and developing recommendations for program improvement based on evaluation findings,
- review evaluation findings and recommendations in regularly scheduled staff meetings,
- engage stakeholders in identifying ways they can apply evaluation findings to improve their programs,
- coordinate, document, and monitor efforts program staff and partners are making to implement improvement recommendations, and
- develop multiple, tailored evaluation reports to address specific stakeholders information needs.

## One Last Note

The impact of the evaluation results can reach far beyond the evaluation report. If stakeholders are involved throughout the process, communication and participation may be enhanced. If an effective feedback loop is in place, program improvement and outcomes may be improved. If a strong commitment to sharing lessons learned and success stories is in place, then other programs may benefit from the information gleaned through the evaluation process. Changes in thinking, understanding, program, and organization may stem from thoughtful evaluative processes (Patton, 2008). Use of evaluation results and impacts beyond the formal findings of the evaluation report start with the planning process and the transparent evaluation plan.

**1** **2** **3** **4** **5** **6**

EVALUATION PLAN TIPS FOR STEP 6

- Planning for use begins with Step 1 and the consideration of stakeholder involvement.
- Evaluation use is likeliest when end use is planned for and built into the six steps in your evaluation plan.
- Use of evaluation is most likely to occur when evaluation is collaborative and participatory, a process that begins in the planning phase.
- An intentional communication and dissemination plan should be included in your evaluation plan.
- The planning stage is the time for the program to begin to think about the best way to share the lessons you will learn from the evaluation.
- In addition to your final report, you will want to tailor reports to highlight specific findings for selected groups of stakeholders. Consider the audience in terms of timing, style, tone, message source, method, and format. Planning for these reports begins with your evaluation plan.

EVALUATION TOOLS AND RESOURCES FOR STEP 6:

- 6.1 Reporting Checklist Exercise
- 6.2 Communicating Results Exercise
- Western Michigan University, The Evaluation Center at http://www.wmich.edu/evalctr/checklists

*AT THIS POINT IN YOUR PLAN, YOU HAVE—*

- *identified the primary users of the evaluation,*
- *created the evaluation stakeholder workgroup,*
- *defined the purposes of the evaluation,*
- *described the program, including context,*
- *created a shared understanding of the program,*
- *identified the stage of development of the program,*
- *prioritized evaluation questions and discussed feasibility issues,*
- *discussed issues related to credibility of data sources,*
- *identified indicators and/or performance measures linked to chosen evaluation questions,*
- *determined implementation roles and responsibilities for program staff, evaluation staff, contractors, and stakeholders,*
- *developed a work plan methods grid,*
- *addressed possible threats to the credibility of your data,*
- *developed a timetable that includes cleaning and analyzing data as well as stakeholder interpretation sessions,*
- *developed an intentional, strategic communications and dissemination plan, and*
- *planned for various audience-specific evaluation reports, presentations, and publications.*

# PULLING IT ALL TOGETHER

Thus far we have walked through the six steps of the CDC Framework for Program Evaluation in Public Health to facilitate programs and their evaluation workgroups as they think through the process of planning evaluation activities. We have described the components of an evaluation plan and details to consider while developing the plan in the context of the CDC Framework. In this section, we briefly recap information that you should consider when developing your evaluation plan.

Increasingly, a multi-year evaluation plan is required as part of applications for funding or as part of program work plans. An evaluation plan is more than a column added to the program work plan for indicators. These plans should be based on stated program objectives and include activities to assess progress on those objectives. Plans should include both process and outcome evaluation activities.

As previously discussed, an evaluation plan is a written document that describes how you will monitor and evaluate your program, so that you will be able to describe the *"What,"* the *"How,"* and the *"Why It Matters"* for your program. The *"What"* reflects the description and accomplishments of your program. Your plan serves to clarify the program's purpose, anticipated expectations, and outcomes. The *"How"* answers the question, "How did you do it?" and assesses how a program is being implemented and if the program is operating with fidelity to the program protocol. Additionally, the *"How"* answers program course-corrections that should be made during implementation. The *"Why It Matters"* represents how your program makes a difference and the impact is has on the public health issue being addressed. Being able to demonstrate that your program has made a difference can be critical to program sustainability. An evaluation plan is similar to a program work plan in that it is a roadmap and is used to guide the planning of activities used to assess the processes and outcomes of a program. An effective evaluation plan is a dynamic tool that can change over time, as needed, to reflect program changes and priorities. An evaluation plan creates directions for accomplishing program goals and objectives by linking evaluation and program planning.

Ideally, program staff, evaluation staff, and the ESW will be developing the evaluation plan while the program is developing the program work plan. Developing the evaluation plan simultaneously with the program work plan allows program staff and stakeholders to realistically think through the process and resources needed for the

> Ideally, program staff and the ESW will develop the evaluation plan while developing the program work plan.

evaluation. It facilitates the link between program planning and evaluation and ensures creating a feedback loop of evaluation information for program improvement and decision making.

Often, programs have multiple funding sources and thus may have multiple evaluation plans. Ideally, your program will develop one overarching evaluation plan that consolidates all activities and provides an integrated view of program assessment. Then, as additional funding sources are sought and activities added, those evaluation activities can be enfolded into the larger logic model and evaluation scheme.

The basic elements of an evaluation plan include:

- Title page
- Question overview
- Intended use and users
- Program description
- Evaluation focus
- Methods
- Analysis and interpretation plan
- Use, dissemination, and sharing plan

However, your plan should be adapted to your specific evaluation needs and context. Additionally, it is important to remember that your evaluation plan is a living, dynamic document designed to adapt to the complexities of the environment within which your programs are implemented. The plan is a guide to facilitate intentional decisions. If changes are made, they are documented and done intentionally with a fully informed ESW.

**Title page:** This page provides easily identifiable program name, dates covered, and possibly basic focus of the evaluation.

**Question overview:** In an evaluation plan, this is an overview of the evaluation questions for ease of reference, similar to the executive summary in a final evaluation report.

**Intended use and users:** This section fosters transparency about the purposes of the evaluation and who will have access to evaluation results. It is important to build a market for evaluation results from the beginning. This section identifies the primary intended users and the ESW and describes the purposes and intended uses of the evaluation.

**Program description:** This section provides a shared understanding of the description of your program and a basis for the evaluation questions and prioritization. This section will usually include a logic model and a description of the stage of development of the program in addition to a narrative description. This section can also facilitate completing the introduction section for a final report or publication from the evaluation. This section might also include a reference section or bibliography related to your program description.

**Evaluation focus:** There are never enough resources or time to answer every evaluation question. Prioritization must be collaboratively accomplished based on the logic model/ program description, the stage of development of the program, program and stakeholder priorities, intended uses of the evaluation, and feasibility issues. This section will clearly delineate the criteria for evaluation prioritization and will include a discussion of feasibility and efficiency.

**Methods:** This section covers indicators and performance measures, data sources and selection of appropriate methods, roles and responsibilities, and credibility of evaluation information. This section will include a discussion about appropriate methods to fit the evaluation question. An evaluation plan methods grid is a useful tool for transparency and planning.

**Analysis and interpretation plan:** Who will get to see interim results? Will there be a stakeholder interpretation meeting or meetings? It is critical that your plans allow time for interpretation and review from stakeholders (including your critics) to increase transparency and validity of your process and conclusions. The emphasis here is on justifying conclusions, not just analyzing data. This is a step that deserves due diligence in the planning process. The propriety standard plays a role in guiding the evaluator's decisions in how to analyze and interpret data to assure that all stakeholder values are respected in the process of drawing conclusions. A timeline that transparently demonstrates inclusion of stakeholders facilitates acceptance of evaluation results and use of information.

**Use, dissemination, and sharing plan:** Plans for use of evaluation results, communications, and dissemination methods should be discussed from the beginning. This is a critical but often neglected section of the evaluation plan. A communication plan that displays target audience, goals, tools, and a timeline is helpful for this section.

The exercises, worksheets, and tools found in Part II of this workbook are to help you think through the concepts discussed in Part I. These are only examples. Remember, your evaluation plan(s) will vary based on program and stakeholder priorities and context.

# REFERENCES

Centers for Disease Control and Prevention. Comprehensive Cancer Control Branch Program Evaluation Toolkit. Atlanta (GA): U.S. Department of Health and Human Services, Centers for Disease Control and Prevention, National Center for Chronic Disease Prevention and Health Promotion, Division of Cancer Prevention and Control, 2010 [accessed 2011 Oct 19].

Centers for Disease Control and Prevention. Framework for Program Evaluation in Public Health. Morbidity and Mortality Weekly Report 1999; 48(NoRR-11):1–40.

Centers for Disease Control and Prevention. Introduction to Process Evaluation in Tobacco Use Prevention and Control. Atlanta (GA): U.S. Department of Health and Human Services, Centers for Disease Control and Prevention, National Center for Chronic Disease Prevention and Health Promotion, Office on Smoking and Health, 2008 [accessed 2011 Oct 19].

Knowlton LW, Philips CC. The Logic Model Guidebook: Better Strategies for Great Results. Thousand Oaks (CA): Sage Publications, 2009.

Lavinghouze R, Price AW, Smith K-A. The Program Success Story: A Valuable Tool for Program Evaluation. Health Promotion Practice 2007; 8(4):323–331.

National Institute on Disability and Rehabilitation Research. Developing an Effective Dissemination Plan. Austin (TX): Southwest Educational Developmental Laboratory, 2001[accessed 2011 Oct 24].

Patton MQ. Utilization-Focused Evaluation. 4th ed. Thousand Oaks (CA): Sage Publications, 2008.

Sandars JR, The Joint Committee on Standards for Educational Evaluation. The Program Evaluation Standards. 2nd ed. Thousand Oaks (CA): Sage Publications, 1994.

Torres R, Preskill H, Piontek ME. Evaluation Strategies for Communicating and Reporting. 2nd ed. Thousand Oaks (CA): Sage Publications, 2004.

Western Michigan University. The Evaluation Center. Evaluation Checklists [accessed 2011 Oct 19].

Worthen BR, Sanders JR, Fitzpatrick JL. Program Evaluation: Alternative Approaches and Practical Guidelines. 2nd ed. New York: Addison Wesley Logman, 1997.

# Part II: Exercise, Worksheets, and Tools

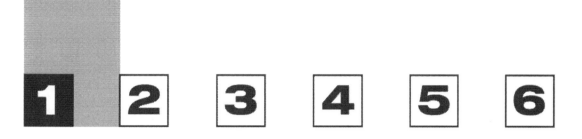

## STEP 1: 1.1 STAKEHOLDER MAPPING EXERCISE

It is suggested that the program enlist the aid of an evaluation stakeholder workgroup (ESW) of 8 to 10 members that represents the stakeholders who have the greatest stake or vested interest in the evaluation.* These stakeholders/primary intended users will serve in a consultative role on all phases of the evaluation. To begin the process of selecting those members who will best represent your primary intended users, it is suggested that you make a list of all possible users with corresponding comments about their investment in the evaluation and potential uses for evaluation results.

| Priority | Person/Group | Comments |
|---|---|---|
|  |  |  |
|  |  |  |
|  |  |  |
|  |  |  |
|  |  |  |
|  |  |  |
|  |  |  |
|  |  |  |
|  |  |  |

*Centers for Disease Control and Prevention. Introduction to Process Evaluation in Tobacco Use Prevention and Control. Atlanta (GA): U.S. Department of Health and Human Services, Centers for Disease Control and Prevention, National Center for Chronic Disease Prevention and Health Promotion, Office on Smoking and Health, 2008 [accessed 2011 Oct 19].

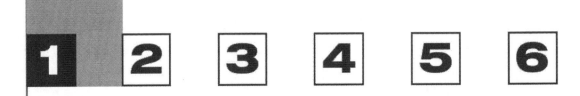

Now, go back over your list of potential users of the evaluation results and consider their level of priority on the list. For example, providing the information that funders or decision makers need may take a higher priority over some clients even though the clients are still very important. You might rate stakeholders in terms of "high," "medium," or "low" or you might rank order them in numerical order (i.e. from "1" to "n"). The choice is yours.

Another method for determining priority users or stakeholders is to conduct a *stakeholder mapping* exercise such as the one that follows. For this activity, choose the characteristics that would be the most beneficial for your evaluation stakeholder group members to have related to their intended use of evaluation results. These characteristics would be the ones determined by the program's staff to be of the most value to your program's evaluation. Write the desired characteristics on the top (Characteristic X) and left-hand side (Characteristic Y) of a 4 x 4 table. Also write whether these characteristics are of high and low value to the program. Characteristics might include traits such as ability to use information, influence over program's future, and direct investment in the program. The traits must be meaningful to the stated purposes of the evaluation.

**Characteristic X**

|  | High | Low |
|---|---|---|
| **High** |  |  |
| **Low** |  |  |

**Characteristic X**

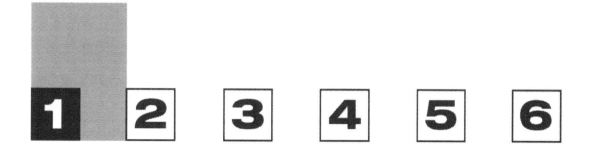

Consider each stakeholder relevant to the evaluation and his or her potential role in the evaluation. Rank the potential evaluation stakeholder as either high or low for each characteristic. Place the stakeholder in the cell that fits his or her importance level for each characteristic.

Characteristic X

|  |  | High | Low |
|---|---|---|---|
| Characteristic X | High | Stakeholder A, B, C, E, G, I, K, M | Stakeholder D, F |
|  | Low | Stakeholder H, J | Stakeholder L, N |

The stakeholders that fall into the high box for both characteristics X and Y would most likely be strong candidates to be invited to be a part of the 8 to 10 person ESW. As with any stakeholder group membership, potential participation would still include additional conversations by program staff.

| Priority | Person/Group | Comments |
|---|---|---|
| | | |
| | | |
| | | |
| | | |
| | | |
| | | |
| | | |
| | | |
| | | |
| | | |
| | | |
| | | |
| | | |
| | | |
| | | |
| | | |
| | | |
| | | |
| | | |
| | | |

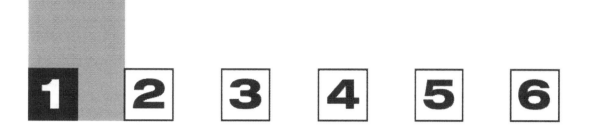

Characteristic X

High                    Low

Characteristic X

High

Low

## STEP 1: 1.2 EVALUATION PURPOSE EXERCISE

As important as identifying the end users and ESW is identifying the **purpose of the evaluation**. These two aspects of the evaluation serve as a foundation for evaluation planning, focus, design, and interpretation and use of results. The purpose of an evaluation influences the identification of stakeholders for the evaluation, selection of specific evaluation questions, and the timing of evaluation activities. It is critical that the program is transparent about intended purposes of the evaluation. If evaluation results will be used to determine whether a program should be continued or eliminated, stakeholders should know this up front.

In order to determine the evaluation purpose, the evaluation team should work with those who are requesting the evaluation to identify the possible multiple purposes for the evaluation from multiple sources. The first task is to consider what groups are interested in an evaluation of the program. This might include the program staff, health department staff, funders, state level decision makers, and other stakeholders. The second task would be to align the specific group with what they are requesting to be evaluated. The next task would be to ascertain what the potential uses of the evaluation results will be by each group interested in the evaluation. And fourth, the team should develop a purpose statement relevant to each group and evaluation requested.

| Group Interested in an Evaluation | What Is to Be Evaluated | How Will the Results Be Used | Evaluation Purpose Statement |
|---|---|---|---|
|  |  |  |  |
|  |  |  |  |
|  |  |  |  |
|  |  |  |  |
|  |  |  |  |

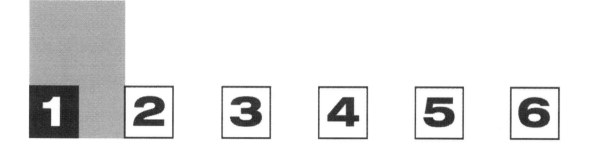

Next, the team should consider each purpose statement for duplication and overlap. What statements could be combined? The final step in the process is to merge the statements into one overall purpose statement.

**Evaluation Purpose Statement:**

| Group Interested in an Evaluation | What Is to Be Evaluated | How Will the Results Be Used | Evaluation Purpose Statement |
|---|---|---|---|
| | | | |
| | | | |
| | | | |
| | | | |
| | | | |
| | | | |
| | | | |
| | | | |

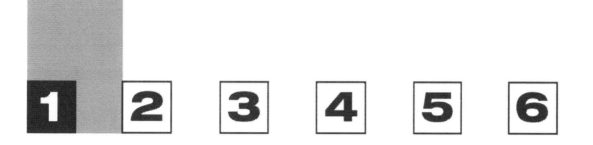

## STEP 1: 1.3 STAKEHOLDER INCLUSION AND COMMUNICATION PLAN EXERCISE

It is important to explore agendas at the beginning of the evaluation and come to a shared understanding of roles and responsibilities as well as the purposes of the evaluation. Some stakeholders will be represented on the ESW and some will not. It is important to include a clear communication plan in your evaluation plan in order to meaningfully engage all appropriate stakeholders and increase participation and buy-in for the evaluation as well as use of final results.

List the appropriate role for each stakeholder relevant to the evaluation and how and when you might engage him or her in the evaluation. It is important to consider a stakeholder's expertise, level of interest, and availability when developing the communication plan. If there are specific deadlines for information such as a community vote or funding opportunity, it is important to note those as well. Additional columns could be added for comments.

| Evaluation Stakeholder | Role Related to the Evaluation | Mode of Communication | Timing of Communication |
|---|---|---|---|
|  |  |  |  |
|  |  |  |  |
|  |  |  |  |
|  |  |  |  |
|  |  |  |  |

A note on roles: Stakeholders need not be a member of the ESW in order to have a role related to the evaluation. Given a stakeholder's specific expertise, interest, availability, or intended use of the evaluation results, he or she may be involved in part or all of the evaluation without being a specific member of the ESW. Roles might include but are not limited to:

- Development of the evaluation plan
- Feedback on focusing the evaluation
- Needing information about specific evaluation activities or progress of the evaluation
- Facilitating implementation of specific aspects of the evaluation
- Participation in interpretation meetings
- Disseminating and promoting use of evaluation results

**1** **2** **3** **4** **5** **6**

| Evaluation Stakeholder | Role Related to the Evaluation | Mode of Communication | Timing of Communication |
|---|---|---|---|
|  |  |  |  |
|  |  |  |  |
|  |  |  |  |
|  |  |  |  |
|  |  |  |  |
|  |  |  |  |
|  |  |  |  |
|  |  |  |  |

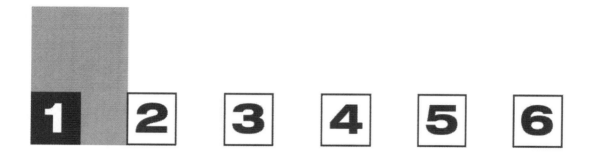

## STEP 1: 1.4 STAKEHOLDER INFORMATION NEEDS EXERCISE

While focusing the evaluation occurs in Step 3, the groundwork begins with the identification of stakeholders relevant to the evaluation or the primary intended users. The ESW membership is designed to reflect the priority information needs of those members who will use the evaluation information. However, it is not always possible to include some high information need groups, and it is certainly not possible to include representation from every group that would benefit from evaluation results. This should not prevent evaluation staff and the ESW from considering all points of view and needs for information when considering how best to focus the evaluation. Therefore, determining stakeholder information needs is both useful for considering membership in the ESW (Step 1) and focusing the evaluation (Step 3).

From your list of primary intended users (those who have a stake in the evaluation results), identify what information each stakeholder will use.

| Primary Intended User (Stakeholder) | Evaluation Information Needed |
|---|---|
| 1. | |
| 2. | |
| 3. | |
| 4. | |
| 5. | |
| 6. | |
| 7. | |
| 8. | |
| 9. | |
| 10. | |
| 11. | |
| 12. | |
| 13. | |
| 14. | |
| 15. | |

| Primary Intended User (Stakeholder) | Evaluation Information Needed |
|---|---|
| 1. | |
| 2. | |
| 3. | |
| 4. | |
| 5. | |
| 6. | |
| 7. | |
| 8. | |
| 9. | |
| 10. | |
| 11. | |
| 12. | |
| 13. | |
| 14. | |
| 15. | |
| 16. | |
| 17. | |
| 18. | |
| 19. | |
| 20. | |

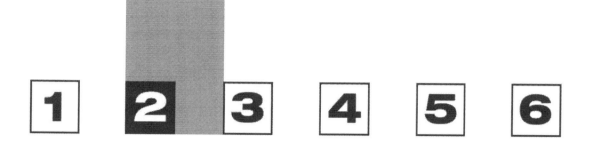

## STEP 2: 2.1 PROGRAM STAGE OF DEVELOPMENT EXERCISE

Another activity that will be needed to fully describe your program and prepare you to focus your evaluation (Step 3) is an accurate assessment of the stage of development of the program. The developmental stages that programs typically move through are **planning, implementation, and maintenance**. It is essential to identify the appropriate stage of development in preparation for focusing the evaluation because some evaluation questions cannot be answered until a program reaches a specific stage of maturation. Stakeholders need to be aware of what the evaluation can and cannot promise. Additionally, preparation for future and sometimes complex evaluations needs to occur in early stages of development for the evaluation to be fully successful.

The stage of development conceptual model is complementary with the logic model. Figure 3.1 shows how general program evaluation questions are distinguished by both logic model categories and the developmental stage of the program. This places evaluation within the appropriate stage of program development (planning, implementation, and maintenance). The model offers suggested starting points for asking evaluation questions within the logic model while respecting the developmental stage of the program. This will prepare the program and the ESW to focus the evaluation appropriately based on program maturity and priorities.

Figure 3.1: Stage of Development by Logic Model Category

| Developmental Stage | Program Planning | Program Implementation | Program Maintenance |
|---|---|---|---|
| **Logic Model Category** | Inputs and Activities | Outputs and Short-term Outcomes | Intermediate and Long-term Outcomes |

To determine what stage of development your program is currently in, staff and stakeholders should have a conversation about program maturation with the logic model in hand. It is important to note that when a program is reinventing itself or revitalization is occurring, the program may resemble the left-hand side of the logic model and thus the program planning stage even when it has been in existence for numerous years.

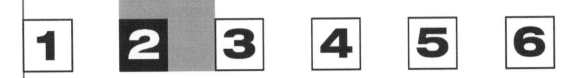

Describe your program's maturation:

| Activities/Tasks That Have Been Completed | Activities/Tasks Working on: | Activities/Tasks Not Yet Begun | Progress Achieved on Outputs or Outcomes (Indicate if Short, Intermediate, or Long Term) |
|---|---|---|---|
| | | | |
| Based on your description and consideration of the logic model, your program is in what stage of development? | | | |
| | | | |

Here is the example of developmental stages from the workbook:

Figure 3.2: Stage of Development by Logic Model Category Example

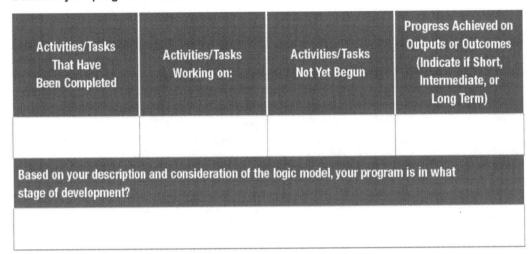

| Developmental Stage | Program Planning | Program Implementation | Program Maintenance |
|---|---|---|---|
| Example: Developmental Stages When Passing a Policy | Assess environment and assets  Develop policy  The policy has not yet been passed | The policy has been passed but not implemented  The policy has been in effect for less than 1 year | The policy has been in effect for 1 year or longer |
| Example: Questions Based on Developmental Stage When Passing a Policy | Is there public support for the policy?  What resources will be needed for implementation of the policy? | Is there compliance with the policy?  Is there continued or increased public support for the policy?  Are there major exemptions or loopholes to the policy? | What is the health impact of the policy? |

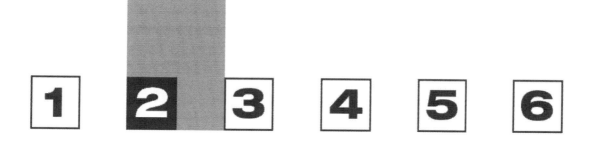

Using the Stakeholder Information Needs chart you prepared in Exercise 1.4, consider the information needed in relation to timing across the logic model. Indicate on this chart what stage of development the program will be in given the nature of the evaluation question asked.

| | Primary Intended User | Evaluation Information Needed | Program Stage of Development |
|---|---|---|---|
| 1. | | | |
| 2. | | | |
| 3. | | | |
| 4. | | | |
| 5. | | | |
| 6. | | | |
| 7. | | | |
| 8. | | | |
| 9. | | | |
| 10. | | | |
| 11. | | | |
| 12. | | | |
| 13. | | | |
| 14. | | | |
| 15. | | | |

What evaluation questions are outside of the current stage of development of your program? What implications does this have for your current evaluation? What implications does this have for planning for future evaluations?

| Activities/Tasks That Have Been Completed | Activities/Tasks Working on: | Activities/Tasks Not Yet Begun | Progress Achieved on Outputs or Outcomes (Indicate if Short, Intermediate, or Long Term) |
|---|---|---|---|
|  |  |  |  |
|  |  |  |  |
|  |  |  |  |
|  |  |  |  |
|  |  |  |  |
|  |  |  |  |

| Based on your description and consideration of the logic model, your program is in what stage of development? |
|---|
|  |

**1** **2** **3** **4** **5** **6**

| Primary Intended User | Evaluation Information Needed | Program Stage of Development |
|---|---|---|
| 1. | | |
| 2. | | |
| 3. | | |
| 4. | | |
| 5. | | |
| 6. | | |
| 7. | | |
| 8. | | |
| 9. | | |
| 10. | | |
| 11. | | |
| 12. | | |
| 13. | | |
| 14. | | |
| 15. | | |
| 16. | | |
| 17. | | |
| 18. | | |
| 19. | | |
| 20. | | |

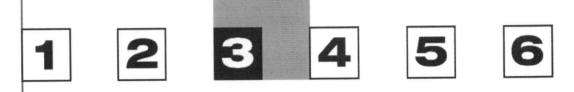

## STEP 3: 3.1 FOCUS THE EVALUATION EXERCISE

The amount of information you can gather concerning your program is potentially limitless. Evaluations, however, are always limited by the number of questions that can be realistically asked, the methods that can actually be employed, the feasibility of data collection, and the available resources. Therefore, the issue at the heart of Step 3 in the CDC framework is focusing the evaluation. The scope and depth of any program evaluation is dependent on program and stakeholder priorities, available resources, including financial resources, staff and contractor availability, and amount of time committed to the evaluation. The program should work together with the ESW to determine the priority of these questions, the feasibility of answering the questions, and identifying the uses of results before designing the evaluation plan.

In this exercise, you will need to consider all the information from previous exercises in Step 1 through Step 2, the logic model, and your stakeholders' vested interest in the evaluation.

From the Stakeholder Mapping exercise, list the stakeholders included in the high-high or priority category for information needs:

| Stakeholders in High-high or Priority Category for Importance and Information Needs |
|---|
|  |
|  |
|  |
|  |
|  |

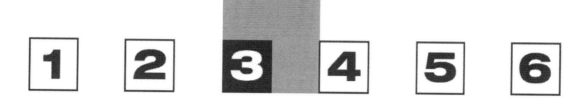

From the Evaluation Purpose Identification exercise, indicate your overall evaluation purpose statement:

| Evaluation Purpose Statement: |
| --- |
|  |

From the Stage of Development exercise, consider each stakeholder's evaluation in relation to the stage of development the program most appropriate for answering that question:

| Primary Intended User | Evaluation Information Needed | Program Stage of Development |
| --- | --- | --- |
| 1. | | |
| 2. | | |
| 3. | | |
| 4. | | |
| 5. | | |
| 6. | | |
| 7. | | |
| 8. | | |
| 9. | | |
| 10. | | |
| 11. | | |
| 12. | | |
| 13. | | |
| 14. | | |
| 15. | | |

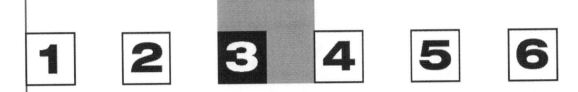

Indicate your program's current stage of development:

| Based on your description and consideration of the logic model, your program is in what stage of development? |
| --- |
|  |

Given the overall purpose statement and the stage of development of the program, what questions from the high-high stakeholder group are viable for the current evaluation effort?

| Evaluation Purpose Statement: | |
| --- | --- |
| Stage of Development of Program: | |
| High-high Category Stakeholders | Evaluation Question |
|  |  |
|  |  |
|  |  |

Next, the team should consider issues of feasibility related to those evaluation questions that are viable options given the current program stage of development and the evaluation purpose.

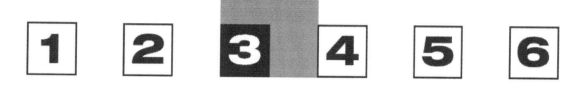

| Evaluation Question | Methods That Might Be Used to Answer the Question | Assumptions or Conditions for This Method to Be Viable | Resources Needed to Implement This Method | Limitations of This Method |
|---|---|---|---|---|
| | | | | |
| | | | | |
| | | | | |
| | | | | |

No chart, grid, or exercise can fully answer the question of how best to focus the evaluation. However, the above information should facilitate informed discussions and can help avoid evaluation activities that are misaligned with the program stage of development, underfunded, or not of the highest priority for information needs. Additional considerations that might help you prioritize your evaluation questions include:

- The questions most important to you and your key stakeholders (the "must answer" questions)
- Questions that provide results that you can use (e.g., for improvement)
- Questions you can answer fully with available or easy to gather data
- Questions within your resources to answer

| The evaluation questions for the current evaluation are: |
|---|
| |
| |
| |
| |

| Evaluation Purpose Statement: | |
|---|---|
| Stage of Development of Program: | |
| High-high Category Stakeholders | Evaluation Question |
| | |
| | |
| | |
| | |
| | |
| | |
| | |
| | |
| | |
| | |

| Evaluation Question | Methods That Might Be Used to Answer the Question | Assumptions or Conditions for This Method to Be Viable | Resources Needed to Implement This Method | Limitations of This Method |
|---|---|---|---|---|
|  |  |  |  |  |
|  |  |  |  |  |
|  |  |  |  |  |
|  |  |  |  |  |
|  |  |  |  |  |
|  |  |  |  |  |
|  |  |  |  |  |

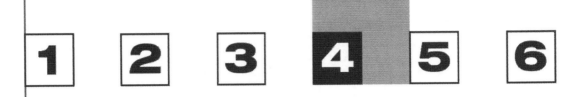

## STEP 4: 4.1 EVALUATION PLAN METHODS GRID EXERCISE

One tool that is particularly useful in your evaluation plan is an **evaluation plan methods grid**. Not only is this tool helpful to align evaluation questions with indicators/performance measures and data sources and roles and responsibilities but it can facilitate advocating for resources for the evaluation. Additionally, this tool facilitates a shared understanding of the overall evaluation plan with stakeholders. This tool can take many forms and should be adapted to fit your specific evaluation and context.

Figure 4.1: Evaluation Plan Methods Grid Example

| Evaluation Question | Indicator/ Performance Measure | Method | Data Source | Frequency | Responsibility |
|---|---|---|---|---|---|
| What process leads to implementation of policy? | N/A | Case study | Site visits and reports | Pre and post funding period | Contractor to be determined |

Figure 4.2: Evaluation Plan Methods Grid Example

| Evaluation Question | Indicators/ Performance Measure | Potential Data Source (Existing/New) | Comments |
|---|---|---|---|
| What media promotion activities are being implemented? | Description of promotional activities and their reach of targeted populations, dose, intensity | Focus group feedback Target Rating Point and Gross Rating Point data sources | |

Choose the grid that is most appropriate for your program and complete it given your chosen evaluation questions from Step 3.

| 1 | 2 | 3 | **4** | 5 | 6 |

| The evaluation questions for the current evaluation are: |
|---|
| |
| |
| |
| |
| |

| Evaluation Question | Indicator/ Performance Measure | Method | Data Source | Frequency | Responsibility |
|---|---|---|---|---|---|
| | | | | | |
| | | | | | |
| | | | | | |
| | | | | | |
| | | | | | |

| Evaluation Question | Indicator/ Performance Measure | Potential Data Source (Existing/New) | Comments |
|---|---|---|---|
| | | | |
| | | | |
| | | | |
| | | | |
| | | | |

Additional possible evaluation plan data grids might look like:

| Evaluation Question | Timeline | Methods | Data Sources | Instruments Needed | Staff/Persons Responsible |
|---|---|---|---|---|---|
|  |  |  |  |  |  |
|  |  |  |  |  |  |

| Evaluation Question | Methods | Instruments Needed | Timeline | Respondents/ Population Sample | Responsibility |
|---|---|---|---|---|---|
|  |  |  |  |  |  |
|  |  |  |  |  |  |

| Evaluation Question | Indicators | Data Collection Sources | Data Collection Methods | Timeline | Data Analysis Plan |
|---|---|---|---|---|---|
|  |  |  |  |  |  |
|  |  |  |  |  |  |

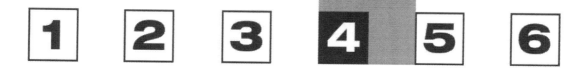

| Evaluation Question | Indicator/ Performance Measure | Method | Data Source | Frequency | Responsibility |
|---|---|---|---|---|---|
| | | | | | |
| | | | | | |
| | | | | | |
| | | | | | |
| | | | | | |
| | | | | | |
| | | | | | |

| Evaluation Question | Indicator/ Performance Measure | Potential Data Source (Existing/New) | Comments |
|---|---|---|---|
| | | | |
| | | | |
| | | | |
| | | | |
| | | | |
| | | | |
| | | | |

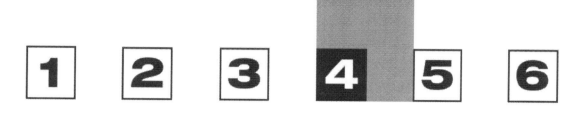

## STEP 4: 4.2 EVALUATION BUDGET EXERCISE

For this exercise, you will need the work plan data grid you completed earlier in Step 4. For this exercise, we have used one as an example, but you should use the one you have chosen as most appropriate for your program.

| Evaluation Question | Indicator/ Performance Measure | Method | Data Source | Frequency | Responsibility |
|---|---|---|---|---|---|
| | | | | | |
| | | | | | |
| | | | | | |
| | | | | | |
| | | | | | |

The team should consider roles and responsibilities, what services might be in kind and what activities will cost additional money. Will you need to pay for additional questions on existing surveys or can you use items that already exist? Are there existing data sources or will you need to create new ones? Do not forget items such as copying costs for surveys or Web services or technology needed in the field, such as recorders or mobile data collection devices.

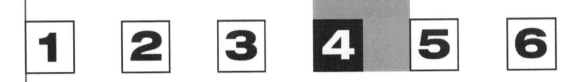

| Evaluation Question | Indicator/ Performance Measure | Method | Data Source | Frequency | Responsibility | Cost Considerations |
|---|---|---|---|---|---|---|
|  |  |  |  |  |  |  |
|  |  |  |  |  |  |  |
|  |  |  |  |  |  |  |
|  |  |  |  |  |  |  |
|  |  |  |  |  |  |  |

Don't be surprised if during this exercise you have to revisit Step 3 or earlier portions of Step 4. Often the budget available doesn't match the evaluation desired. Either the evaluation scope will need to be reduced or additional resources obtained. It is better to thoroughly consider this now before implementation begins than have to change course mid-implementation cycle.

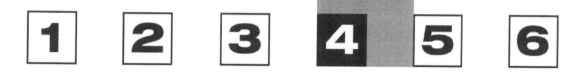

| Evaluation Question | Indicator/ Performance Measure | Method | Data Source | Frequency | Responsibility | Cost Considerations |
|---|---|---|---|---|---|---|
|  |  |  |  |  |  |  |
|  |  |  |  |  |  |  |
|  |  |  |  |  |  |  |
|  |  |  |  |  |  |  |
|  |  |  |  |  |  |  |
|  |  |  |  |  |  |  |
|  |  |  |  |  |  |  |

## STEP 5: 5.1 STAKEHOLDER INTERPRETATION MEETING EXERCISE

Justifying conclusions includes analyzing the information you collect, interpreting what the data mean, and drawing conclusions based on the data. This step is needed to turn the data collected into meaningful, useful, and accessible information. This is often the step in which programs incorrectly assume they no longer need the stakeholder workgroup and that this step is better left to the "experts." However, including your stakeholder group in this step is directly tied to the previous discussion on credibility and acceptance of data and conclusions.

Moreover, it is critical that your plans allow time for interpretation and review from stakeholders (including your critics) to increase transparency and validity of your process and conclusions. The emphasis here is on justifying conclusions not just analyzing data. This is a step that deserves due diligence in the planning process. The propriety standard plays a role in guiding the evaluator's decisions on how to analyze and interpret data to assure that all stakeholder values are respected in the process of drawing conclusions.* This may include one or more stakeholder interpretation meetings to review interim data and further refine conclusions. A note of caution, as a stakeholder-driven process, there is often pressure to reach beyond the evidence when drawing conclusions. It is the responsibility of the evaluator and the evaluation workgroup to ensure that conclusions are drawn directly from the evidence.

---

*Sandars JR, The Joint Committee on Standards for Educational Evaluation. The Program Evaluation Standards. 2nd ed. Thousand Oaks (CA): Sage Publications, 1994.

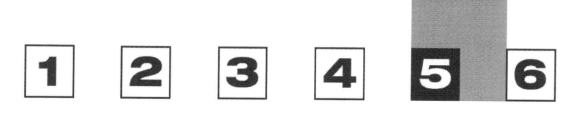

A variety of activities can be included in your evaluation plan to solicit stakeholder input and facilitate interpretation of evaluation data. An example is provided below:

| Interpretation and Review Activities | Timeline |
|---|---|
| Individual site evaluation reports and feedback | Within 1 month of site visit |
| Check-in with ESW and/or participants | Within 3 months of site visit or as appropriate during analysis phase |
| Grantee interpretation meeting | Immediately following preparation of preliminary results |
| Stakeholder interpretation meeting | Within 3 months following the grantee interpretation meeting |
| Stakeholder review of draft final report | Within 3 months following the stakeholder interpretation meeting |
| Clearance and review process of final report | Within 2 months following stakeholder review of draft final report |

Complete an outline of proposed activities appropriate to your evaluation project to include opportunities for stakeholder interpretation and feedback:

| Interpretation and Review Activities | Timeline |
|---|---|
|  |  |
|  |  |
|  |  |
|  |  |
|  |  |
|  |  |

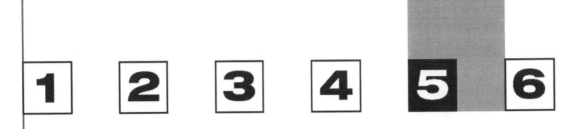

It is important to consider the time it takes to solicit and incorporate stakeholder feedback in your evaluation project timeline. At this time, you should revisit your budget and timeline created earlier to ensure adequate time and funding for the stakeholder inclusion process.

In order to make sure your stakeholder interpretation meeting is a success, plan for steps to help things run smoothly. Time for these activities needs to be included in your evaluation timeline.

- Send the initial invitation at least 2 months in advance so that stakeholders can plan for the meeting. Remind stakeholders of the overall evaluation purpose and questions.
- Send the preliminary report or PowerPoint presentation within 2 weeks of the initial invitation to allow stakeholders time to review. It is important to remind stakeholders that results are a draft and should not be shared outside of the review group.
- Send reminders about the meeting 1 or 2 weeks prior to the date. Identify any pre-existing documentation that may be useful for understanding context.
- Plan for appropriate technology (and backup) needed such as recorders, laptop, and screen, flipcharts.
- If feasible, use a professional meeting facilitator.

A checklist to facilitate the development of a formal stakeholder interpretation meeting can be found at http://www.wmich.edu/evalctr/checklists/checklist_topics/.

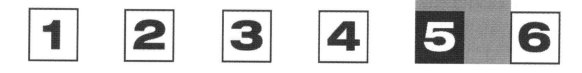

| Interpretation and Review Activities | Timeline |
|---|---|
|  |  |
|  |  |
|  |  |
|  |  |
|  |  |
|  |  |
|  |  |
|  |  |
|  |  |
|  |  |
|  |  |

**1 2 3 4 5 6**

## STEP 6: 6.1 REPORTING CHECKLIST EXERCISE

It may be helpful to include a draft table of contents and outline for sections of the final report in the evaluation plan. Additionally, the team could discuss preliminary ideas for tailored evaluation reporting and include these ideas in the dissemination plan. Below is a checklist of items that may be worth discussing during the evaluation planning stage to ensure adequate time and resources are devoted to the implementation and reporting process.

## Tools and Templates: Checklist for Ensuring Effective Evaluation Reports*

- ☐ Provide interim and final reports to intended users in time for use.
- ☐ Tailor the report content, format, and style for the audiences by involving audience members.
- ☐ Include an executive summary.
- ☐ Summarize the description of the stakeholders and how they were engaged.
- ☐ Describe essential features of the program (e.g., in appendices).
- ☐ Explain the focus of the evaluation and its limitations.
- ☐ Include an adequate summary of the evaluation plan and procedures.
- ☐ Provide all necessary technical information (e.g., in appendices).
- ☐ Specify the standards and criteria for evaluative judgments.
- ☐ Explain the evaluative judgments and how they are supported by the evidence.
- ☐ List both strengths and weaknesses of the evaluation.
- ☐ Discuss recommendations for action with their advantages, disadvantages, and resource implications.
- ☐ Ensure protections for program clients and other stakeholders.
- ☐ Anticipate how people or organizations might be affected by the findings.
- ☐ Present minority opinions or rejoinders where necessary.
- ☐ Verify that the report is accurate and unbiased.
- ☐ Organize the report logically and include appropriate details.
- ☐ Remove technical jargon.
- ☐ Use examples, illustrations, graphics, and stories.

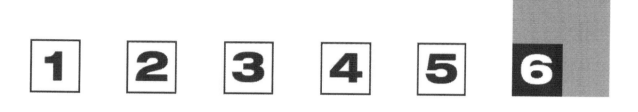

*Adapted from Worthen BR, Sanders JR, Fitzpatrick JL. Program Evaluation: Alternative Approaches and Practical Guidelines. 2nd ed. New York: Addison Wesley Logman, 1997; presented in Centers for Disease Control and Prevention. Comprehensive Cancer Control Branch Program Evaluation Toolkit. Atlanta (GA): U.S. Department of Health and Human Services, Centers for Disease Control and Prevention, National Center for Chronic Disease Prevention and Health Promotion, Division of Cancer Prevention and Control, 2010 [accessed 2011 Oct 19].

Also visit The Evaluation Center at Western Michigan University online for a free evaluation report checklist:

http://www.wmich.edu/evalctr/checklists/checklist_topics/.

# 1 2 3 4 5 6

## STEP 6: 6.2 COMMUNICATING RESULTS EXERCISE

Your evaluation results may not reach the intended audience with the intended impact just because they are published. An intentional communication and dissemination plan should be included in your evaluation plan. As previously stated, the planning stage is the time for the program to address the best way to share the lessons you will learn from the evaluation. The communication-dissemination phase of the evaluation is a two-way process designed to support use of the evaluation results for program improvement and decision making. In order to achieve this outcome, a program must translate evaluation results into practical applications and must systematically distribute the information or knowledge through a variety of audience-specific strategies.

Communicating evaluation results involves sharing information in ways that make it understandable and useful to stakeholders. Successful communication is key to your evaluation results being used. You can do this by using a variety of communication formats and channels. A communication format is the actual layout of the communication you will use, such as reports, brochures, one-page descriptions, newsletters, executive summaries, slides, and fact sheets. A communication channel is the route of communication you will use, such as oral presentations, videos, e-mails, webcasts, news releases, and phone conferences. Both the formats and channels should take into account the needs of different audiences, the type of information you wish to provide, and the purpose of the communication.

When developing your communication or dissemination strategy, carefully consider the following:

- With which target audiences or groups of stakeholders will you share findings?
- What formats and channels will you use to share findings?
- When and how often do you plan to share findings?
- Who is responsible for carrying out dissemination strategies?

You can use the following matrix to help you plan your communication process.

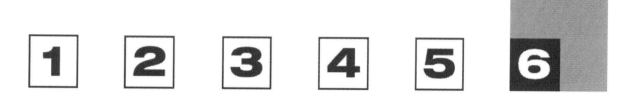

| What do you want to communicate? | To whom do you want to communicate? | How do you want to communicate? | |
| --- | --- | --- | --- |
| | | Format(s) | Channel(s) |
| | | | |
| | | | |
| | | | |
| | | | |

** This tool was adapted from DASH's Communication Matrix in Using Evaluation to Improve Programs: Strategic Planning in the Strategic planning kit for school health programs. Available at: http://www.cdc.gov/healthyyouth/evaluation/sp_toolkit.htm [accessed 2011 Oct 19].

This tool can help you track communications with your various audiences, including the communication format(s) (the layout of the communication, such as newsletters) and the communication channel(s) (the route of communication, such as oral presentations), audience feedback on the communication message, and next steps you need to take in response.

| Communication | Date | Communication Format(s) | Communication Channel(s) | Audience Feedback and Next Steps |
| --- | --- | --- | --- | --- |
| | | | | |
| | | | | |
| | | | | |

A second example of a tracking chart might look like this:

| Target Audience (Priority) | Objectives for the Communication | Tools | Timetable |
|---|---|---|---|
|  |  |  |  |
|  |  |  |  |
|  |  |  |  |
|  |  |  |  |
|  |  |  |  |

Here is the example from the workbook:

Figure 5: Communication Plan Table

| Target Audience (Priority) | Goals | Tools | Timetable |
|---|---|---|---|
| Program Implementation Team | Inform them in real time about what's working well and what needs to be quickly adjusted during implementation | Monthly meetings and briefing documents | Monthly |
| Program Stakeholders | Promote program progress | Success stories | Annually |
| Funding Decision Makers | Continue and/or enhance program funding | Executive summary; Targeted program briefs | Within 90 days of conclusion of funding |

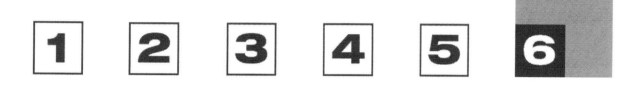

| What do you want to communicate? | To whom do you want to communicate? | How do you want to communicate? | |
|---|---|---|---|
| | | Format(s) | Channel(s) |
| | | | |
| | | | |
| | | | |
| | | | |
| | | | |
| | | | |
| | | | |

**1** **2** **3** **4** **5** **6**

| Communication | Date | Communication Format(s) | Communication Channel(s) | Audience Feedback and Next Steps |
|---|---|---|---|---|
| | | | | |
| | | | | |
| | | | | |
| | | | | |
| | | | | |
| | | | | |
| | | | | |
| | | | | |

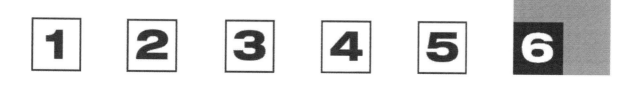

| Target Audience (Priority) | Objectives for the Communication | Tools | Timetable |
|---|---|---|---|
| | | | |
| | | | |
| | | | |
| | | | |
| | | | |
| | | | |
| | | | |

## OUTLINE: 7.1 BASIC ELEMENTS OF AN EVALUATION PLAN

Often, programs have multiple funding sources and, thus, may have multiple evaluation plans. Ideally, your program will develop one overarching evaluation plan that consolidates all activities and provides an integrated view of program assessment. Then, as additional funding sources are sought and activities added, those evaluation activities can be enfolded into the larger logic model and evaluation scheme.

Your plan should be adapted to your specific evaluation needs and context. Additionally, it is important to remember that your evaluation plan is a living, dynamic document designed to adapt to the complexities of the environment within which your programs are implemented. The plan is a guide to facilitate intentional decisions. If changes are made, they are documented and done intentionally with a fully informed ESW.

The basic elements of an evaluation plan include:

- Title page
- Question overview
- Intended use and users
- Program description
- Evaluation focus
- Methods
- Analysis and interpretation plan
- Use, dissemination, and sharing plan

## OUTLINE: 7.2 EVALUATION PLAN SKETCHPAD

Often, groups do not have the luxury of months to develop an evaluation plan. In many scenarios, a program team has only one opportunity to work with their ESW to develop their evaluation plan to submit with a funding proposal. All of the work discussed in this workbook must be accomplished in a single workgroup meeting, retreat, or conference session. In this scenario, it is helpful to have an evaluation sketchpad to develop the backbone or skeleton outline of your evaluation plan. With the major components of your evaluation plan developed, you will have the elements necessary to submit a basic evaluation plan that can be further developed with your funder and future stakeholders. Even if you have time to fully develop a mature evaluation plan, this sketchpad exercise is often a great tool to use to work with an ESW in a retreat type setting.

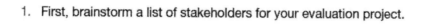

1. First, brainstorm a list of stakeholders for your evaluation project.

| Priority | Person/Group | Comments |
|---|---|---|
| | | |
| | | |
| | | |
| | | |
| | | |
| | | |
| | | |
| | | |
| | | |
| | | |
| | | |

2. Go back to your list and circle high-priority stakeholders or high-priority information needs.

From the list of high-priority stakeholders identified above, think about their information needs from the evaluation or about the program.

| Primary Intended User | Information Needed |
|---|---|
| 1. | |
| 2. | |
| 3. | |
| 4. | |
| 5. | |
| 6. | |
| 7. | |
| 8. | |
| 9. | |

Discuss the intended uses of the evaluation by primary intended users and program staff:

| Primary Intended User/Program Staff | Intended Uses |
|---|---|
| 1. | |
| 2. | |
| 3. | |
| 4. | |
| 5. | |
| 6. | |
| 7. | |
| 8. | |
| 9. | |

3. Discuss potential political agendas or environmental constraints (Hidden agendas—from stakeholders, team members, company). What goals and objectives for the evaluation do stakeholders come to the table with before you even begin the evaluation? What is most important to each of the stakeholders at the table?

| Stakeholder | Goals/Objectives |
|---|---|
| | |
| | |
| | |
| | |
| | |
| | |
| | |
| | |
| | |

4. Briefly describe your program (in your plan you will include your logic model(s) if you have one):

| Description of Program: |
|---|
| |

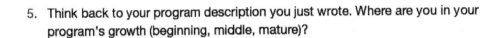

5. Think back to your program description you just wrote. Where are you in your program's growth (beginning, middle, mature)?

| Stage of Growth: |
| --- |
|  |

6. Based on where you are in your program's growth, what does that tell you about what kinds of questions you can ask?

| Stage of Growth | Questions |
| --- | --- |
| Beginning |  |
| Middle |  |
| Mature |  |

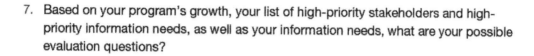

7. Based on your program's growth, your list of high-priority stakeholders and high-priority information needs, as well as your information needs, what are your possible evaluation questions?

| Your evaluation questions for the current evaluation are: |
| --- |
|  |
|  |
|  |
|  |

8. Now, take each question and think about ways you might answer that question. Will your method be qualitative, quantitative or both? Do you already have a data source? Will you have some success stories? How much will it cost? What resources do you have? Who needs to be involved to make the evaluation a success? How will you ensure use of lessons learned? How and when will you disseminate information? Below are two samples of tables you can use to organize this information.

| Evaluation Question | Indicator/ Performance Measure | Method | Data Source | Frequency | Responsibility |
|---|---|---|---|---|---|
| | | | | | |
| | | | | | |
| | | | | | |
| | | | | | |
| | | | | | |
| | | | | | |
| | | | | | |
| | | | | | |

| Evaluation Question | Indicator/ Performance Measure | Method | Data Source | Frequency | Responsibility | Cost Considerations |
|---|---|---|---|---|---|---|
| | | | | | | |
| | | | | | | |
| | | | | | | |
| | | | | | | |
| | | | | | | |
| | | | | | | |
| | | | | | | |

9. Now think about the different ways you might communicate information from the evaluation to stakeholders. Communication may include information to stakeholders not on your ESW. You may want to provide preliminary results, success stories, etc. throughout the evaluation. Additionally, your ESW may assist in your communication efforts. What deadlines must be met and what opportunities are lost if deadlines are not met. How will this impact the timetable you created in #8?

| What do you want to communicate? | To whom do you want to communicate? | How do you want to communicate? | |
| --- | --- | --- | --- |
| | | Format(s) | Channel(s) |
| | | | |
| | | | |
| | | | |
| | | | |
| | | | |
| | | | |
| | | | |

# LOGIC MODEL EXAMPLES
## OSH Logic Models Example

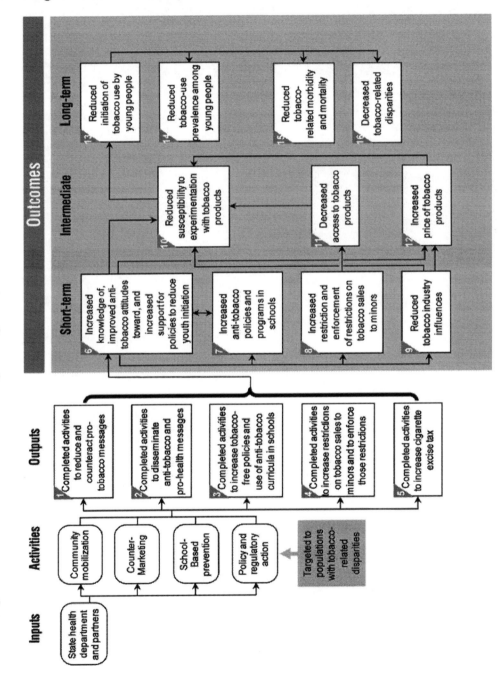

Preventing Initiation of Tobacco Use Among Young People

Eliminating Nonsmokers' Exposure to Secondhand Smoke

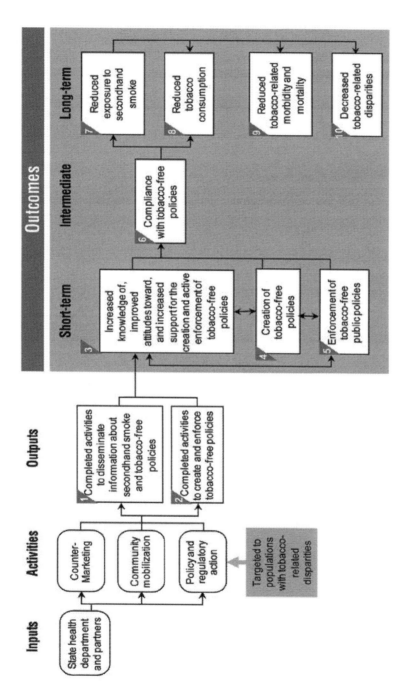

Promoting Quitting Among Adults and Young People

Figure: Logic model for Promoting Quitting Among Adults and Young People

**Inputs**
- State health department and partners

**Activities**
- Counter-marketing
- Community mobilization
- Policy and regulatory action

Targeted to populations with tobacco-related disparities

**Outputs**
1. Completed activities to disseminate information about cessation
2. Cessation quitline is operational
3. Completed activities to work with health care systems to institutionalize PHS-recommended cessation interventions
4. Completed activities to support cessation programs in communities, workplaces, and schools
5. Completed activities to increase insurance coverage for cessation interventions
6. Completed activities to increase tobacco excise tax

**Outcomes**

*Short-term*
7. Establishment or increased use of cessation services
8. Increased awareness, knowledge, intention to quit, and support for policies that support cessation
9. Increase in the number of health care providers and health care systems following Public Health Service (PHS) guidelines
10. Increased insurance coverage for cessation services

*Intermediate*
11. Increased number of quit attempts and quit attempts using proven cessation methods
12. Increased price of tobacco products

*Long-term*
13. Increased cessation among adults and young people
14. Reduced tobacco-use prevalence and consumption
15. Reduced tobacco-related morbidity and mortality
16. Decreased tobacco-related disparities

# DNPAO Logic Model Example

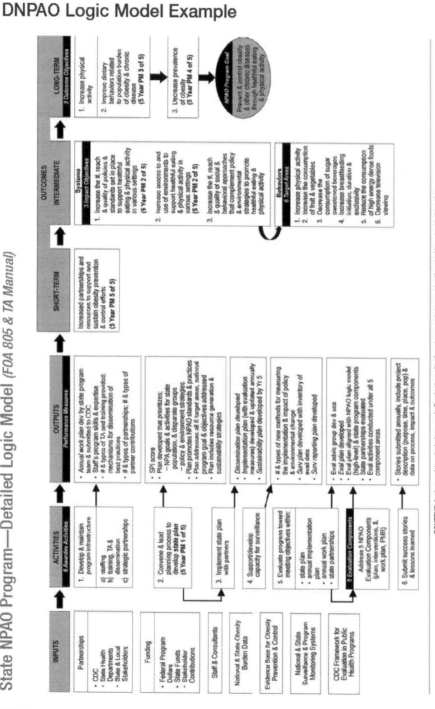

State NPAO Program—Detailed Logic Model *(FOA 805 & TA Manual)*

# Resources *

*Resources are listed for the convenience of the user and do not constitute endorsement by the U.S. Government.

## WEB RESOURCES

**American Evaluation Association**

- http://www.eval.org/
- The American Evaluation Association (AEA) is an international professional association of evaluators devoted to the application and exploration of program evaluation, personnel evaluation, technology, and many other forms of evaluation. Evaluation involves assessing the strengths and weaknesses of programs, policies, personnel, products, and organizations to improve their effectiveness. AEA has approximately 5,500 members representing all 50 states in the United States as well as over 60 foreign countries. [accessed 2011 Jul 19]

**Centers for Disease Prevention and Control (CDC) Division of Adolescent and School Health's Program Evaluation Resources and Tools**

- http://www.cdc.gov/healthyyouth/evaluation/resources.htm

**CDC Division of Sexually Transmitted Disease Prevention's Practical Use of Program Evaluation among Sexually Transmitted Disease (STD) Programs**

- http://www.cdc.gov/std/program/pupestd/Introduction-SPREADS.pdf

**CDC Framework for Program Evaluation**

- http://www.cdc.gov/eval/framework/index.htm
- Effective program evaluation is a systematic way to improve and account for public health actions that involve procedures that are useful, feasible, ethical, and accurate. The framework guides public health professionals in their use of program evaluation. It is a practical, nonprescriptive tool, designed to summarize and organize essential elements of program evaluation. The framework comprises steps in program evaluation practice and standards for effective program evaluation. Adhering to the steps and standards of this framework will allow an understanding of each program's context and will improve how program evaluations are conceived and conducted.

**CDC Introduction to Program Evaluation for Public Health Programs: A Self Study Guide**

- http://www.cdc.gov/getsmart/program-planner/downloads/Manual_04062006.pdf

**Disseminating Program Achievements and Evaluation Findings to Garner Support**

- http://www.cdc.gov/healthyyouth/evaluation/pdf/brief9.pdf

**Impact and Value: Telling Your Program's Story**

- http://www.cdc.gov/oralhealth/publications/library/success_stories_wkbk.htm

**National Heart Disease and Stroke Prevention Program's Evaluation Guides: Writing SMART Objectives; Developing and Using Logic Models**

- http://www.cdc.gov/dhdsp/programs/nhdsp_program/evaluation_guides/logic_model.htm

**Penn State Extension Program Evaluation Resources**

- http://extension.psu.edu/evaluation/

**Western Michigan University: The Evaluation Center**

- http://www.wmich.edu/evalctr/checklists/

- This site provides refereed checklists for designing, budgeting, contracting, staffing, managing, and assessing evaluations of programs, personnel, students, and other evaluations; collecting, analyzing, and reporting evaluation information; and determining merit, worth, and significance. Each checklist is a distillation of valuable lessons learned from practice.

**University of Wisconsin Extension: Program Development and Evaluation publications**

- http://www.uwex.edu/ces/pdande/evaluation/evaldocs.html

- This site provides a range of publications for planning and implementing an evaluation and offers online evaluation curriculums and courses.

**W.K. Kellogg Foundation: Logic Model and Development Guide**

- http://www.wkkf.org/knowledge-center/resources/2006/02/WK-Kellogg-Foundation-Logic-Model-Development-Guide.aspx

- A guide to logic modeling to facilitate program planning and implementation activities.

## MAKING YOUR IDEAS STICK, REPORTING, AND PROGRAM PLANNING

Atkinson C. Beyond Bullet Points: Using Microsoft Office PowerPoint 2007 to Create Presentations That Inform, Motivate, and Inspire. Microsoft Press, 2007.

Becker HS. Writing for Social Scientist: How to Start and Finish Your Thesis, Book, or Article. Chicago, IL: University of Chicago Press, 2077, 2nd ed.

Heath C, Heath, D. Made to Stick: Why some Ideas Survive and Others Die. New York, NY: Random House, 2007.

Heath C, Heath D. Switch: How to Change Things When Change is Hard. New York, NY: Random House, 2010.

Impact and Value: Telling Your Program's Story

- www.cdc.gov/oralhealth/publications/library/success_stories_wkbk.htm

Lavinghouze R, Price AW, Smith, KA. The Program Success Story: A Valuable Tool for Program Evaluation. Health Promotion Practice, 2007; 8(4): 323–331.

Torres R, Preskill H, Piontek ME. Evaluation Strategies for Communicating and Reporting. Thousand Oaks, CA: Sage Publications, Inc., 2004, 2nd ed.

## QUALITATIVE METHODS

Miles MB, Huberman, MA. Qualitative Data Analysis. Thousand Oaks, CA: Sage Publications, Inc., 1994, 2nd ed.

Patton M.Q. Qualitative Research and Evaluation Methods. Thousand Oaks, CA: Sage Publications, Inc., 2001, 3rd ed.

Yin RK. Case Study Research: Design and Methods (Applied Social Research Methods) Thousand Oaks, CA: Sage Publications, Inc., 2008, 4th ed.

Yin RK. Qualitative Research from Start to Finish. New York, NY: The Guilford Press, 2010.

## QUANTITATIVE METHODS

Kleinbaum DG, Klein M. Logistic Regression: A Self-Learning Text (Statistics for Biology and Health. Springer, New York, NY, 2010, 3rd ed.

Rothman KJ, Greenland S, Lash TL. Modern Epidemiology. Philadelphia, PA: Lippincott Williams & Wilkins, 2008, 3rd ed.

Tufte ER. Envisioning Information. Cheshire, CT: Graphics Press, 1990.

Tufte ER. The Visual Display of quantitative Information. Cheshire, CT: Graphics Press, 2001.

## EVALUATION USE

Butterfoss FD. Coalitions and Partnerships in Community Health. San Francisco, CA: Jossey-Bass, 2007.

Mattessich PW. The Manager's Guide to Program Evaluation: Planning, Contracting, and Managing for Useful Results. St. Paul, Minnesota: Amherst H. Wilder Foundation, 2003.

Patton MQ. Developmental Evaluation: Applying Complexity Concepts to Enhance Innovation and Use. New York, NY: The Guilford Press, 2010.

Patton MQ. Utilization-Focused Evaluation. Thousand Oaks, CA: Sage Publication, 2008, 4th ed.

## OSH EVALUATION RESOURCES

**Best Practices for Comprehensive Tobacco Control Programs—2007**

- http://www.cdc.gov/tobacco/stateandcommunity/best_practices/index.htm
- *CDC's Best Practices for Comprehensive Tobacco Control Programs—2007* is an evidence-based guide to help states plan and establish effective tobacco control programs to prevent and reduce tobacco use.

**Evaluation Toolkit for Smoke-Free Policies**

- http://www.cdc.gov/tobacco/basic_information/secondhand_smoke/evaluation toolkit/index.htm
- The evaluation approaches described in this toolkit and the findings of studies conducted using these approaches may also be useful to stakeholders who are interested in the effects of smoke-free laws, including business organizations (e.g., chambers of commerce, restaurant associations) and labor unions.

### Introduction to Process Evaluation in Tobacco Use Prevention and Control

- www.cdc.gov/tobacco/tobacco_control_programs/surveillance_evaluation/process_evaluation/index.htm

- Published in 2008, this guide will help state and federal program managers and evaluation staff design and implement valid, reliable process evaluations for tobacco use prevention and control programs.

### Introduction to Program Evaluation for Comprehensive Tobacco Control Programs

- http://www.cdc.gov/tobacco/tobacco_control_programs/surveillance_evaluation/evaluation_manual/index.htm

- Published in 2001, this "how to" guide for planning and implementing evaluation activities will help state tobacco control program managers and staff in the planning, design, implementation, and use of practical and comprehensive evaluations of tobacco control efforts.

### Key Outcome Indicators for Evaluating Comprehensive Tobacco Control Programs

- http://www.cdc.gov/tobacco/tobacco_control_programs/surveillance_evaluation/key_outcome/index.htm

- Published in 2005, this guide provides information on 120 key outcome indicators for evaluation of statewide comprehensive tobacco prevention and control programs.

### Question Inventory on Tobacco (QIT)

- http://apps.nccd.cdc.gov/qit/quickSearch.aspx

- This Web-based tool developed by CDC's Office on Smoking and Health categorizes more than 6,000 tobacco-related questions. This site can be used to collect information on survey questions used in the past, locate available data for secondary analyses, and gather ideas for future instrument development.

### Quitlines: A Resource for Development, Implementation, and Evaluation

- http://www.cdc.gov/tobacco/quit_smoking/cessation/quitlines/index.htm

- This 2005 document is intended to help state health departments, health care organizations, and employers to contract for and monitor telephone-based tobacco cessation services. It is also designed to help states, health care organizations, and quitline operators enhance existing quitline services and to inform those who are interested in learning more about population-based approaches to tobacco cessation.

**Smoking—Attributable Mortality, Morbidity, and Economic Costs (SAMMEC)**

- http://apps.nccd.cdc.gov/sammec/

- This online application allows you to estimate the health and health-related economic consequences of smoking to adults and infants.

**State Tobacco Activities Tracking and Evaluation (STATE) System**

- http://www.cdc.gov/tobacco/statesystem

- The STATE System is an electronic data warehouse containing up-to-date and historical state-level data on tobacco use prevention and control.

**Surveillance and Evaluation Data Resources for Comprehensive Tobacco Control Programs**

- http://www.cdc.gov/tobacco/tobacco_control_programs/surveillance_evaluation/ surveillance_manual/index.htm

- Published in 2001, this compilation of data sources for tobacco control programs is useful for tobacco control programs that are conducting surveillance or evaluation.

**Surveillance and Evaluation Net-Conferences**

- Archived presentations available at: http://www.ttac.org/resources/cdc_ netconferences.html

- The Surveillance and Evaluation Net-conference series provides information on evaluation best and promising practices and describes the role of evaluation in tobacco control work. The Net-conference series was originally designed for state surveillance and evaluation staff, but the material covers a variety of interesting and emerging topics in surveillance and evaluation that are valuable to other public health professionals. Each conference consists of a lecture followed by a question and answer session.

**Surveillance and Evaluation Web page on CDC-OSH's Smoking and Tobacco Use website**

- http://www.cdc.gov/tobacco/tobacco_control_programs/surveillance_evaluation/ index.htm

**Tobacco Control State Highlights 2010**

- http://www.cdc.gov/tobacco/data_statistics/state_data/state_highlights/2010/index.htm

- Tobacco Control State Highlights 2010 guides states in developing and implementing high-impact strategies and assessing their performance. This report also provides state-specific data intended to—highlight how some states are making great strides in reducing smoking rates using evidence-based strategies while also showing that more work needs to be done in other states, enable readers to see how their own states perform, and help policymakers with decision making.

# DNPAO EVALUATION RESOURCES

### Developing and Using an Evaluation Consultation Group

- http://www.cdc.gov/obesity/downloads/EvaluationConsultationGroup.pdf
- An Evaluation Consultation Group (ECG) is required for all state obesity programs funded by the Division of Nutrition, Physical Activity and Obesity (DNPAO) to provide technical, programmatic, and related input to the program evaluation of the state health department's NPAO work. This guidance provides a systematic approach to evaluating an ECG including a series of steps and tools for conducting the evaluation.

### Evaluation of State Nutrition, Physical Activity, and Obesity Plans

- www.cdc.gov/obesity/downloads/EvaluationofStateNPAOPlans.pdf
- This guide clarifies approaches to and methods of evaluation; provides examples and tools specific to the scope and purpose of state nutrition, physical activity and obesity programs; and recommends resources for additional reading.

### Evaluation: Quick Start Resources

- http://www.cdc.gov/nccdphp/dnpa/physical/pdf/PA_evaluation_quick_start.pdf
- This resource provides a list of key references and tools for planning and implementing program and/or project evaluations, focusing specifically on physical activity programs and evaluations.

### Recommended Community Strategies and Measurements to Prevent Obesity in the United States

- http://www.cdc.gov/mmwr/preview/mmwrhtml/rr5807a1.htm
- This report identifies and recommends a set of 24 strategies and associated measurements that communities and local governments can use to plan and monitor environmental and policy-level changes for obesity prevention.

National Center for Chronic Disease Prevention and Health Promotion

18144488R00066

Made in the USA
Middletown, DE
29 November 2018